PARLIAMENTS AND SCREENING

Collection Éthique et Science
under the direction of Gérard Huber

PARLIAMENTS AND SCREENING

A CONFERENCE ON THE ETHICAL
AND SOCIAL PROBLEMS ARISING
FROM TESTING AND SCREENING FOR HIV
AND AIDS : THE ROLE OF PARLIAMENTS
AND THE MEDIA

CONFERENCE REPORT
AND
STUDIES OF THE HANDLING OF BIOETHICS
IN THE TWELVE NATIONAL PARLIAMENTS
OF THE EUROPEAN UNION

Edited by
Wayland Kennet
in association, for the conference,
with Paul Robinson

ASSOCIATION DESCARTES

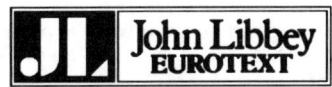

British Library Cataloguing in Publication Data
A catalogue record for this book is available from the British Library.

ISBN 2-7420-0095-X

Éditions John Libbey Eurotext
127, avenue de la République, 92120 Montrouge, France
Tél. : (1) 46.73.06.60

John Libbey & Company Ltd
13, Smiths Yard, Summerley Street,
London SW18 4HR, England
Tel. : (1) 947.27.77

John Libbey CIC
Via L. Spallanzani, 11
00161, Rome, Italy
Tel.: (06) 862.289

‡ John Libbey Eurotext, Paris, 1995

Il est interdit de reproduire int-gralement ou partiellement le pr-sent ouvrage — loi du 11 mars 1957 — sans autorisation de l'-diteur ou du Centre Fran"ais du Copyright, 6 bis, rue Gabriel-Laumain, 75010 Paris, France.

CONTENTS

Preface: W. Kennet 1

Part one
Conference report

Introduction: W. Kennet 9
The ethics of testing and screening for HIV: J. Harris, R. Bennet 15
Common law chaos: screening for HIV: M. Brazier ... 29
Discussion 40

Genetic screening-1: P. Nairne 59
Genetic screening-2: C. Miles 65
Invited response: L. Honnefelder 71
Discussion 72

The role of the media: J. Durant, A. Hansen 89
Invited response: J. Maddox 107
Discussion 109

Legislation and regulation in Europe: experience and prospect: W. Kennet 123
The role of parliaments: W. Kennet, L. Kluver 137
Discussion 140

Short presentations by relevant intergovernmental organizations: S.S. Fluss, G. Kutukdjian, A. Isola, J. Elizalde 147
Invited contribution: C. Campbell 155
Discussion 157

The future: general discussion 165

VI PARLIAMENTS AND SCREENING

Part two
Bioethical information in the national parliaments of the European Union

Introduction: W. Kennet 171

Bioethics and the Belgian Parliament: G. Binamé 173

Bioethical information in the Danish Parliament: B.A. Rix 183

Bioethics in the French Parliament: B. Rullier 197

Structure and processes of information acquisition in the German Parliament: AIDS and « Genetic Engineering/Genetic Testing »: T. Petermann, E. Göll 221

The means of information available to the Hellenic Chamber of Deputies on matters of bioethics: S.I. Koutsoubinas 245

Bioethical information in the Irish Parliament: V. ni Bhroinn 253

Bioethics in the Italian Parliament: S. Rodota 261

Biotechnology and the Luxembourg Parliament: F. Cocard 265

Providing the Netherlands Parliament with information on normative aspects of screening and testing for HIV and genetic diseases: G.M.W.R. de Wert, I. Ravenschlag, M.A.M. de Wachter 269

Bioethics in the Portuguese Parliament: A. Martins, J. Leitao 301

Bioethics in the Spanish Parliament: M. Palacios 309

Bioethics information in the United Kingdom Parliament: P. Davis 317

Conclusion: W. Kennet 335

List of participants 343

Preface

The programme

Under its programme of biomedical research BIOMED 1, the European Commission in 1993 entered into a contract with the Descartes Society of Paris (Association Descartes). This is a Society devoted to increasing the public understanding of science in France, and is one hundred percent Government funded. Its offices are in the Ministry of Research and Higher Education.

Under the contract, the Society has set up and managed a programme called: "Bioethics in Europe: Survey, Analysis and Information." This programme was to run for three years: 1993-1995. Projects were set up in five Member Sates of the European Union as follows: France, led by Dr Gérard Huber, the Secretary of the Descartes Society; Germany, led by Dr Stella Reither-Theil of Gottingen University; Italy, led by Professor Stefano Rodota, Professor of Law in the University of Rome, and then a member of the Italian Parliament; the Netherlands, led by Dr Maurice de Wachter of the Institute of Bioethics at Maastricht; and the United Kingdom, led by Lord Kennet, a member of the House of Lords. These five people collectively constituted the Management Board of the Project, which usually meets in Paris, but sometimes in the other cities concerned.

Each of these five people agreed to prepare and convene a conference, and to produce a book arising from the conference and its constituent papers. The conferences were to be as follows:

1. London, January 1994, on Parliaments and screening for HIV and genetic disease, convened by Lord Kennet: the conference which gives rise to this book.

2. Maastricht, June 1994, on Euthanasia and assisted suicide convened by Dr Maurice de Wachter.

3. Rome, December 1994, on the Private sphere and genetics, convened by Professor Stefano Rodota.

4. Paris, May 1995, Ethics and therapy for human brain disease and psychic disorders, convened by Dr Gérard Huber.

5. September 1995, on Informed consent in psychiatry, convened by Dr Stella Reiter-Theil.

As this book goes to press, the first three conferences have been held.

The London Conference

The Conference was held in London on January 20th and 21st 1994, and was concerned with the relation between, on the one hand, the social and ethical consequences of the recent headlong advances in molecular biology, and, on the other, the national Parliaments of Europe which must either legislate to regulate them, or consciously refrain from doing so.

To bring the subject within the bounds of a two day meeting, the conference was limited to the social and ethical consequences of testing and screening for HIV and for genetic disease, and the roles of Parliament and the news media in that matter.

The major funding for the London Conference was from Directorate General XII of the European Commission (Science

Research and Development) under the Descartes Society contract, and from Directorate General V of the Commission (Health and Safety). There were also minor but most helpful grants from the Wellcome Trust of London, a major medical foundation; Zeneca plc, a major British bio-corporation; and from the Economic and Social Research Council, which is funded by the British Government.

The conference was held in association with the Parliamentary and Scientific Committee. This Committee, founded in 1939, is the main interface in the United Kingdom between Parliament and the worlds of science and technology. Its membership consists of some two hundred members of both Houses, most British universities, many scientific learned associations, and about eighty high-tech companies. It holds meetings and conferences, and publishes a periodical: *Science in Parliament*. Sir Gerard Vaughan, MP, who was then the Chairman of the Committee, chaired one of the conference sessions; Lord Kennet is a Vice-President of the Committee.

The conference was held in the house of the Royal Society in London. The Royal Society corresponds to the National Academy of Science in other countries. It was founded in 1660 by King Charles II. Sir Isaac Newton, who was also a Member of Parliament, was its President from 1703-1727.

The first session, on HIV testing, was organized jointly with the Centre for Social Ethics and Policy in the University of Manchester, which was at the time engaged in a separate project on the ethics of HIV screening, funded by DG XII.

The second session was organized jointly with the Nuffield Council on Bioethics of London. This Council was set up in 1991, at the suggestion of the Government, to consider the problems of bioethics in much the same way as the national ethics committees do in those countries which have them. It had recently completed its first report, on genetic testing, and this conference was the first international discussion of that report.

Participation in the conference was by invitation. People were invited from every country then in the Union, and a few from other European countries. One hundred and sixteen came, of whom fifty seven were British, and fifty nine were from other countries or from international organizations. Among them were thirteen members of parliaments, four parliamentary officials, and many who are called on by governments and parliaments for advice. A list is at Appendix A.

The twelve parliaments study

The conference had before it not only the prepared papers of the principal speakers, but also the Five Parliaments Study. This consisted of reports on the way five European national parliaments handle bioethics and information about bioethics. It consisted of a bound booklet which was circulated in advance to the participants of the Conference, and wider. It constituted the first tranche of the Twelve Parliaments Study. The latter was completed during 1994, and makes up the second part of this book.

The book

This book is published by John Libbey Eurotext, who is the official publisher to the Descartes Society. Its publication has been made possible by a separate grant from DG XII of the European Commission.

The organizers wish to thank all the funders of the Conference and of the book, on behalf of all those who have contributed to either. As convener and editor, I wish to thank the Royal Society, the Parliamentary and Scientific Committee, the Nuffield Council on Bioethics, and the Centre for University of Manchester Department of Applied Philosophy for the work they put into the project. I thank the Descartes Society, with mixed surprise and pleasure, for having allowed me to undertake this rewarding work in the first place. And with especial warmth, I thank those who contributed the separate national papers to the Twelve Parliaments Study for their patience and care in following a plan which was of varying degrees of relevance to their respective countries.

Wayland Kennet

Part one

CONFERENCE REPORT

Introduction

WAYLAND KENNET[1]

This is a conference largely about Parliaments, and my original intention was — an intention laid up in heaven — that there should be a good scattering of Parliamentarians from all the Community national Parliaments here. But this is a difficult week for our Parliaments, even more difficult than usual, which is saying a lot, since there is no profession in the world where it is harder to make an appointment in advance and then actually be free to keep it. It is a plenary session week for the European Parliament; the French Parliament is actually in special session this week, debating bioethics with an unprecedented emphasis and publicity; the Italian Parliament is in a special position in the run up to the next elections, which I do not think anybody is unaware of; and even our own Parliament is having a pretty tense time, though not as tense as the Italian.

This conference is part of a series organized by the Descartes Society of Paris. I have a message from Professor François Gros, the president of that Society, wishing us well in our work, and another from Dr. Gérard Huber, who is the secretary of the Society and the chairman of the International Manage-

---

1. Vice-President, the Parliamentary and Scientific Committee. Formerly British Government Minister and MEP.

ment Committee of the whole project of which we form part; he is unfortunately unwell, so I shall read his message to you.

"I am most grateful for your kind invitation to say a few words in this most prestigious house. I would first like to address you my sincere congratulations on the conception of such an original conference, based on the comparison between different perceptions of testing and screening for HIV and genetic diseases. As the chairman of the Management Group of the Concerted Action 'Bioethics in Europe: Survey, Analysis and Information', I wish to thank the whole Group which has helped you in the task of deepening this concept. At this very point in time in France, Parliament is debating a bill on bioethics. This explains the absence of Professor Mattei, who is in charge of it for the French Government. I also wish to convey the apologies of Professor Francois Gros, who is the president of the Descartes Society and the Scientific Adviser to Commissioner Ruberti, and whose responsibilities in the Académie des Sciences prevent him from joining us today.

Everybody knows the ancient Greek tradition which formally distinguishes between opinion and knowledge. Bioethics has to pass from the first to the second, that is to say from a bioethics exclusively based on subjective judgement, to another one based on objective judgement. Now this target will not be attained if we do not rise above the level of method to the level of the methodology of research into bioethics. Methodology is our main expert tool: that is why our group has put forward the inventory and comparative analysis of the specific decisions taken by the actors in the field of biomedicine and society, at whatever decision level, in the name of bioethics. You have chosen both the parliamentary and the media levels. I am sure that it is a good choice, because the members of the national and the European Parliaments will have the opportunity to exchange informations about their respective practices, at least as far as bioethics is concerned. Moreover, society does not know the methods used by Parliaments to take decisions in their name in the field of bioethics.

INTRODUCTION
11

By way of conclusion, I am happy to announce that our team will set up a group specifically about the methodology of research into bioethics. I remain sure it is a most successful event."

Professor Andersen has kindly agreed to chair our first session in the place of Mme Noelle Lenoir, the chairman of the UNESCO International Bioethics Committee, who has been prevented from coming because of a meeting of the French Council of State, of which she is also a Member.

I turn now to the substance of our meeting.

What is screening? This is our first question. Who screens whom, and what for, and on what basis of existing information, with what intentions, with what degree of accuracy, and by whom is that accuracy judged? We shall examine that today: first the established practice of HIV testing, and then the nascent one of genetic testing and screening.

On our second day, we shall turn to political issues, otherwise known as issues of public ethics: what Parliaments do, might do and should do about biomedical developments, and how the press goes about its business reporting and commenting on them. Screening opens up possible conflicts between public health aims and individual welfare and rights. At the individual level, what is the effect of HIV screening, and what may be the effect of genetic screening not only on a person's self but on her baby, other members of her family, descendants, sexual partners: all this we have to go into. We shall also, I hope, touch on the question of genetic fingerprinting.

At the level of society: what are the social problems which face Governments and Parliaments in regulating, or arranging for the regulation of testing and screening and of the information they yield? The Council of Europe has made a most useful distinction between five types of screening:

— voluntary,
— systematic offered (offered to all persons in some category),
— systematic anonymous (as above, but the tests to be anonymous),
— mandatory as a condition for voluntary activities (for instance, blood donation and volunteers for military service), and lastly,
— compulsory for all.

Are there subdivisions for these categories?

We shall go on to consider screening for genetic diseases, which is becoming rapidly established in our countries: how do these two cases fit in the context of democratic management of issues of biomedical ethics in general?

There is a spectrum of intervention by public power running from statute and secondary law, through the appointment of regulating bodies by Parliaments and the legal endorsement of professional self-regulation, down to the most tentative guidelines which may be drawn up by hospital ethics committees for their own use. Since the art of politics is to take good decisions on inadequate evidence, legislators have to consider not only the quality of the information being presented to patients, but also of the information on which they, the legislators, have to act. Hypotheses, evidence, conclusions, forecasts, particularly of timescales: the whole spectrum of the possible.

In any particular case, is something science produces hard enough and suggestive enough of risk for this to be the right time for the State to act? That is a very different question from whether it is the right time for the caring professions to act. Problems for legislators might include not only the quality of the information at any time on the grounds of which irreversible treatment may either be offered or not, but also the distinction between on the one hand bringing the disadvantaged or ill up to average health, and on the other hand improving the general health of a people, and what the latter might mean.

Next, the role of the media — tomorrow morning. Legislators, if they are not in the first place driven by public opinion, must carry public opinion with them. They must also face the problem of public misinformation by the media and by pundits. In a free society, the media report or misreport, inform or misinform, and respect or invade privacy pretty much as they please, and no information can be exempt from media criticism solely because Governments and Parliaments believe it is true and it is vital that people should have access to it. Is public misinformation about HIV different from other public information because HIV kills? How should this problem be considered by Governments, Parliaments and the media themselves?

Lastly, our Parliamentary session. Law and regulation have grown up in the European Community more or less without co-ordination among the member states: did this matter? The balance between legislation and professional regulation varies from country to country. Does the existence of the single market make it expedient to seek harmonization in the materials or procedures used in screening? Here the question of patents arises, which we are not considering in this conference, but which certainly deserves careful examination.

We have carried out a comparative study recording the means by which national Parliaments in the European Community inform themselves on bioethical matters with a view to legislation. It was distributed to you in advance. We may next ask ourselves, what if any, attention should be paid to the diffusion of genetic screening technologies to countries with less stable or less liberal forms of government than the Western democracies, and to the formation of opinion in those countries? The shadow of eugenics in Germany and in the United States in the 1930s forces the questions. All these things I hope we shall discuss.

The ethics of testing and screening for HIV

JOHN HARRIS[1], REBECCA BENNET[2]

The first question this paper must answer is why test and screen for HIV at all? Without a cure for AIDS, we must rely on prevention based on education. Accurate information about the spread of the virus is clearly a necessary part of a successful AIDS prevention campaign, allowing appropriate preventative and therapeutic measures to be developed. Such information would enable evaluation of the effectiveness of existing health education programmes and allow authorities to plan the required health care provision. Good information will increasingly enable the targeting of effective public health measures and help combat prejudice and popular misconceptions. The testing of individuals would allow those at risk to receive appropriate counselling and treatment. Which raises the question of mandatory testing.

Mandatory testing?

There is no doubt that medical, therapeutic and scientific research on AIDS is in the public interest. The research not

---
1. Professor of Applied Philosophy, Research Director of the Center for Social Ethics and Policy, University of Manchester.
2. Research Fellow of the same Center.

only benefits ourselves but also future generations. Although we recognize an individual's general right to privacy or control of information about himself, in some circumstances, it is clear that these rights are outweighed by the possibility of preventing disease or premature death in countless present and future people who might benefit.

If you are inclined to doubt this, consider:

The ship in distress. If a ship's captain diverts his passenger ship into a storm to go to the aid of a stricken vessel, he puts his passengers at some extra risk to their lives and certainly, will knowingly subject them to anxiety, distress and even pain and injury. The risks will of course vary, but they may be substantial. If the seas are very rough, minor injuries from falls and so on may be almost inevitable. His justification is surely that he must weigh against the extra risks to his passengers the fact that others will certainly lose their lives if they are not rescued. It is generally accepted that captains of ships have both a right and a duty to act in this way[3].

If the information generated by testing and screening is important for preventing the spread of HIV, it might be argued that almost any measures that would provide the most extensive statistical data available, should be adopted. It might, therefore, be suggested that a system of universal mandatory testing should be introduced.

Yet mandatory testing has been unequivocally rejected by the Council of Europe[4] and the World Health Organization and is arguably not only expensive and impractical, but also offensive. But of course it might be that we should offend in a good cause.

Ethically, mandatory testing poses many complex problems. It challenges personal autonomy and violates the right of all

---

3. See Harris J. *Wonderwoman and Superman: The Ethics of Human Biotechnology.* Oxford University Press, Oxford, 1992, Chapter 5.
4. See Council of European Committee of Ministers Recommendation No. R (87) 25 to the Member States concerning a common European Public Health policy to fight the Acquired Immunodeficiency Syndrome (AIDS), 26 November 1987.

citizens to refuse medical touchings, a right which is legally protected in many jurisdictions. However, we should be wary of basing our objections to mandatory testing on the right to refuse the laying on of medical hands, in short, on the right not to be assaulted. While at the moment tests for HIV require blood samples which in turn require the invasion of bodily integrity to retrieve the sample, it may be that, in the future, such tests will be possible via, say, a sample of saliva retrievable from deposits on a drinking glass. If this becomes possible, such samples might be taken surreptitiously without the necessity of obtaining consents and hence bypass legislative constraints on assault and battery.

In addition to these ethical considerations, mandatory testing would seem unworkable on a practical level. As HIV tests normally test for the anti-bodies to the virus and not for the virus itself, and it can take up to three to four months for antibodies to develop, it is possible for an individual to receive a negative result when he is in fact already HIV seropositive. For mandatory testing to provide anything like an accurate picture of the extent of infection in a population, HIV tests would have to be repeated at least every three months.

Far from having to accept difficult and extreme measures which seriously violate a persons' autonomy it may be that the civil rights of an individual are entirely compatible with, and even essential to, an effective HIV prevention strategy. As has been argued: It is our intuition that we should think in terms of reciprocity of obligations, that is, in terms of a reciprocity between obligations *to* the seropositive individual and obligations *of* the seropositive individual. It should be confirmed that the HIV seropositive individuals be treated with the respect they are due as persons, and that they remain fully integrated within society and are not ostracized, stigmatized or labelled. It would be unrealistic, for example, to hope for HIV seropositive individuals' serious recognition of a duty to disclose their serostatus if to do so is to open those individuals to discrimination[5].

---

5. The Center for Social Ethics and Policy, "AIDS: Ethics, Justice and European Policy", 1992.

An effective HIV/AIDS prevention programme will depend on those who are HIV seropositive and those who have reason to suspect they are HIV seropositive feeling able to come forward and seek advice without the fear of discrimination. This cannot be possible in a context in which hostility, coercion, ignorance and prejudice are rife.

We believe that a system of voluntary testing and screening combined with legislative safeguards against discrimination could provide the statistical information for as effective a preventative strategy as is currently possible, and allow individuals to be tested for HIV anti-bodies without the threat of disastrous consequences.

Anonymous screening

The public interest requires an effective epidemiological surveillance system so that guesstimates can be replaced by properly researched data showing the distribution and extent of the disease. As we have already ruled out universal mandatory testing, it is important to find a way of collecting substantial statistical information whilst allowing for the protection of the autonomy of the individual. A programme of voluntary testing combined with anonymous screening would seem to have the potential for satisfying this criterion.

Anonymous HIV serosurveys, similar to those developed in the United Kingdom, normally involve the testing of blood already taken for other purposes and inevitably involve the testing of specific groups in society; for instance in the United Kingdom such testing involves the testing of patients attending General Practices, Genito-Urinary Medicine (GUM) Clinic Services and hospitals.

Those opposed to this type of screening argue that involuntary screening of this kind entails ethical problems of its own for a number of reasons. Firstly, to carry out the test without the explicit consent of the patient violates autonomy. In addition, it is sometimes felt that health professionals dealing with patients have the right to know the serostatus of their patients in order to protect themselves from infection. Finally, it may be felt that people tested have the right to know the result of the test, especially if the result is positive.

Problems of consent

Consent would normally be needed before testing for HIV anti-bodies and it is generally accepted that counselling and advice should be provided before the test, to ensure that the individual is aware of the possibly distressing consequences of such a test[6].

In the case of anonymous screening, the British Medical Association[7] has argued that, since the information is coded and cannot be traced back to the individual, there cannot be any adverse consequences and so consent would be unnecessary. However, it will be difficult to be completely confident about the anonymity of screening. There will always be a danger of disclosure as long as information is stored. The unacceptability of this danger may be countered by pointing out that the risk of leaks can be justified by the use to which the information can be put to save lives.

Problems of confidentiality. Universal precautions

It should not be necessary, routinely[8], to inform health professionals of positive results gained as a result of an anony-

---

6. Unfortunately, although pre- and post-test counselling should ideally be a priority, such counselling is not always possible. In many non-industrialised countries, although excellent counselling is available, it is not always possible to provide counselling on the scale that is needed.
7. British Medical Association (BMA). "BMA urges anonymous testing". *The Guardian*, 27 August 1988.
8. Except perhaps where health professionals are involved in "risky procedures", for example, some forms of orthopaedic surgery.

mous serosurvey. Health professionals should, as standard practice, protect themselves from HIV and other possible infections as it is impossible to know the serostatus of all patients. There may however be some particularly risky medical procedures where it might be argued that health professionals are entitled to know the HIV status of their patients, though many eloquently deny this. There is, however, a particular problem where safeguards fail and a health professional wants to assess the level of risk. Relaying information about the results of such screening to the individuals concerned, or to health professionals who feel they might be at risk, would involve the same infringements of an individuals autonomy that are apparent with mandatory testing. The patient does not consent to receiving information about his/her HIV status, and certainly has not consented to interested third parties being granted access to this information.

However, if the test is positive, are we not obliged to inform the individual involved of his/her status to enable that individual to receive treatment and counselling and protect those around him/her from infection?

The problem is, of course, that if it became known that, by attending certain medical treatment centres or undergoing certain procedures, you were automatically tested for HIV and informed of any positive results, there might be a danger that people would be reluctant to come forward for treatment at these centres or for those procedures. If these centres included drug rehabilitation and GUM clinics, this deterrent might negate the benefits of screening.

Mandatory tests. Voluntary results

We believe it would be worth considering a screening strategy whereby individuals must consent to anonymous screening where blood is voluntarily given for other purposes, but can also decide whether they wish to know the results of the test or not. In this way, those who may have been dissuaded from coming forward for treatment, through fear of knowing their HIV status, could come forward without apprehension, and it would also be possible, in cases where consent was given, to contact patients who receive a positive result without compromising those persons fundamental rights.

Screening in this way necessarily entails focusing on certain groups in society as a result of individuals seeking specific medical treatment and, as such, is obviously limited in value, as results do not represent a true cross section of society. But as long as individuals are protected against disclosure of information as far as is possible and are only informed of their own HIV status when consent has been given, screening can be a useful source of information without being unethical.

Voluntary testing and justice

We gain little by compromising a person's autonomy in the quest to develop effective preventative strategies in the face of HIV/AIDS. Indeed it might be argued that respect for a person's autonomy and moral rights is an essential tool for the development of effective public health strategies.

Equal respect for the moral rights of all people is central to the notion of justice. As outlined elsewhere: However we may like to conceive of justice, many would now recognize that the principle of equality lies at its core. The ethical principle of equality may be stated briefly: each person within each community is entitled to and should be afforded equal respect, concern, and protection. At the basis of this principle is the idea that persons are of equal importance. Justice, constructed very loosely as fairness, would lack significance if we did not accept that persons matter equally and hence are equally entitled to fair treatment. A consequence of the principle of equality is that we should not discriminate unfairly between individual members or group within a community. In the context of health policy and its reaction to the AIDS pandemic, the principle is vitiated if we do not actively seek to afford all non-infected citizens what protection against infection exists, or if we do not provide HIV seropositive individuals with adequate care of their symptoms, and therapy as and when it becomes available, and protection against unfair discrimination[9].

If social policy in the face of HIV/AIDS was to be constructed in terms of these reciprocal obligations and a commitment to this principle of equality, an environment could be developed in which an HIV seropositive individual would not be subject to the sort of discrimination and fear of discrimination that may deter others from coming forward for testing or forewarning their partners or third parties whom they consider to be at risk of HIV infection.

In the present climate of discrimination, the Terrance Higgins Trust, for example, advises those contemplating a test for HIV to consider whether the benefits are worth the risk. The likely consequences of voluntary testing are that an individual could be in an extremely compromising position was he to take the test. If individual's rights were by contrast protected, the number of people coming forward for testing would gradually increase as confidence in the effectiveness of protection became established. In this way, voluntary testing would provide useful statistical information and those taking the test would receive guidance and advice. Subsequently, public health strategies could be enhanced, not by undermining individual's rights, but by actively enforcing them.

The success or otherwise of such a social policy and any consequent HIV prevention strategy would depend upon the State effectively realizing its obligation to advise and protect persons who are HIV seropositive or have reason to think they might be.

---

9. Erin C.A., Harris J. AIDS: Ethics, Justice and Social Policy. *Journal of Applied Philosophy.*

So-called "innocent and guilty" AIDS victims: responsibility for one's own adverse health state

Fear of possible HIV infection is natural, but when this fear is based on ignorance and prejudice it can be counterproductive to the prevention of infection. By blaming minorities, it may be that we are dissipating these fears by assuring ourselves that it "can't happen to me". We gain a false sense of security which is fuelled by suspicion and hostility of those infected.

The popular view of HIV as a disease mainly affecting homosexual men dramatically increases the potential for discrimination. Homosexuality had been viewed with suspicion long before HIV infection was identified as prevalent in Western gay populations. If our aim is to protect ourselves from infection, hostility and discrimination against those infected is counterproductive quite apart from being offensive. Individuals will be reluctant to come forward for testing and advice if they are likely thereby to experience discrimination and hostility.

If care and protection on the one hand, or priority for treatment on the other, are to vary according to an individual's own responsibility for his/her adverse health state, few would merit care and protection or have anything but a low priority. From cream-cakes to car racing, from smoking to obesity, we are almost all "guilty" to some degree.

It may be argued that the possibility of using information about the HIV status of an individual to disadvantage that individual should be avoided by maintaining the individuals' confidentiality at all costs, guaranteeing information will not pass into the hands of third parties without the consent of the subject.

But such a guarantee would seem to be impossible. If uncoded records are kept, whatever security measures are taken to limit the accessibility, there will always be the possibility of leaks especially when information could have considerable value for others.

There are several senses in which information connected to HIV testing is valuable.

Value to others

Firstly, the information is valuable to others who may wish to protect themselves from infection. We have already argued that health professionals do not normally need to know the serostatus of individuals in order adequately to protect themselves. However, if the information was available it would certainly be obtained with consequent danger of leaks and abuse.

The right of partners of HIV seropositive individuals to be advised of this risk is unarguable. It has been suggested that in cases where HIV infected individuals refuse to inform or protect partners at risk, the need to protect an individuals' right to confidentiality is overridden by the possibility of infecting others.

Commercial value

Information relating to a likely fatal disease will clearly have value relating to cost effectiveness for insurance companies and employers. Insurers and employers may demand information on HIV serostatus as a condition of contract and it would be impossible to block in non-disclosure.

Confidential information of this kind may have commercial value and may be of interest to insurance under writers, employers and even the "gutter" press, as information on HIV status, or even the fact that the test has been taken may be seen to yield further clues about private lives of the famous or notorious.

With value like this and the essentially leaky nature of computer records, there can be no guarantee of confidentiality. With no possibility of absolute confidentiality, the solution must be to protect individuals not from the release of information but at least from some of the worst consequences.

If we accept the principles of equality and justice as fundamental to the functioning of society, it must follow that we should not discriminate unfairly between individual members or groups in the community. To allow individuals who are HIV seropositive or are thought to be at risk from HIV infection to be denied rights that would seem to be central to modern notions of equality such as the right to work, the right to provide for dependants and the right to buy a home, would certainly contravene the principles of most democratic societies.

Right to work

Employers are under a moral obligation within most democratic systems not to discriminate unfairly in the employment opportunities they offer, or to expose employees to unavoidable risk. It follows that an employer would only be justified in excluding an employee on the grounds of HIV status, if the risk that the employee represents to the employer, other employees or third parties is so severe as to justify the consequent discrimination against the employee.

As there is no evidence that HIV is transmitted through normal casual social contact, the likelihood of infection of third parties is very low. In most cases, HIV individual will not represent a risk to colleagues, and if a risk is present it will be minimal, certainly not so significant as to justify discrimination. Very few jobs involve contact with bodily fluids and it would be unacceptable to discriminate against HIV positive individuals in most cases on the surely spurious grounds that they pose a threat to colleagues and others in the course of their work.

Not only is it unacceptable to discriminate against HIV seropositive persons on the grounds that they present a severe risk to others, but it is also unacceptable to discriminate against such individuals on the grounds that it may not be cost-efficient to employ someone with a high likelihood of suffering episodic illness and who ultimately is likely to die very prematurely.

If we think it wrong for an employer to be permitted to discriminate against women on the grounds that they are statistically likely to wish to take time out to have children and that they are consequently less cost effective as employees than men, we do so because we recognize that the right to work, or not to be discriminated against in the provision of employment opportunities is important and the added costs of such a policy are such as should be borne in order to do justice.

Discrimination against particular individuals or particular types of individuals, in the provision of employment is a major wrong, whether that wrong is analyzed in terms of respect for persons, or in terms of violation of their rights [10].

At the moment, there is very little explicit legislation to prevent discrimination against HIV seropositive individuals. In most cases, it is likely that individuals would decide against an industrial tribunal because of fears of publicity and the increased discrimination which could follow. We must, therefore, protect the employees right to work by strengthening existing laws and creating specific legal safeguards to protect those tested for HIV and give effective training and advice to workers in an attempt to allay irrational fears of infection.

Insurance

The issue of AIDS and the issues of surrounding genetic testing and screening lead inexorably to demanding that insurers

---

10. See Harris J., *op. cit.*, Oxford University Press, Oxford, 1992.

act as if they had not more information which is or will be available to them, but no information. We believe we should prevent all insurers from acquiring and using any information, other than the information about the general statistical risks in a population, in other words no personal information at all. Premiums should be set for persons of a particular age, given the general background risks within society.

We believe that in the face of the increasing, and increasingly accurate information that will be available via genetic screening, this is the only way in which many people will be able to be provided fairly with insurance protection in the community. It seems to us that insurers could not be worse off if they apply such a policy since, with the increasingly effective healthcare that screening will enable, the overall health of the community is likely to improve rather than get worse.

Conclusion

To facilitate a strategy of HIV/AIDS prevention based on education, we must focus on social policy which is constructed in terms of a reciprocity between the obligations *to* the seropositive individual and the obligations *of* the seropositive individual. Screening and testing of the kind proposed within a frame work of policy based on this reciprocity of obligations would provide the statistical information for an effective preventative strategy and allow individuals to come forward to receive testing and preventative advice without the fear of disastrous consequences.

The way forward must be to protect individuals, not from the release of information, but at least from some of the worse consequences of disclosure. What is needed is some formal recognition to the right to privacy, combined with specific legislation protecting the fundamental rights of those affected by HIV/AIDS. Effective legislation is needed to allow protection against unfair discrimination which may prohibit individuals from access to insurance, health care, housing and employment. Legislation required would be immensely complex, would probably effect issues of freedom of speech and press, and would have to be carefully thought out, but such legislation must be formulated if we are to facilitate an effective strategy of HIV prevention.

Common law chaos: screening for HIV

MARGARET BRAZIER [1]

I have entitled my paper Common Law Chaos because I believe it is an apt description of the state of legal debate in relation to screening for human immunodeficiency virus (HIV). I must, however, acknowledge that there is not at present hard evidence that anyone is much the worse for this alleged chaos.

It is important to understand first that, in the United Kingdom, the law defining the rights of patients and the professional obligations of health care workers remains largely judge-made law. Judge-made law, the common law, is crucial to any analysis of the law governing screening for HIV. Indeed legislation in relation to HIV at all is minimal in the United Kingdom. Despite its awesome title, the AIDS (Control) Act 1987 simply provides for the compilation of anonymous statistics on the incidence of the disease in this country. The Public Health (Infectious Diseases) Regulations 1988 extend to AIDS provisions of the Public Health Act 1984 providing for the compulsory detention and treatment of people with AIDS. This power of coercive treatment will be discussed more fully later in the paper and has to my knowledge only ever been used on one occasion (in Manchester).

---

1. Professor of Law and Legal Studies, Legal Director of the Centre of Social Ethics and Policy in Manchester University.

The common law thus addresses all the important questions relating to screening, in particular what constitutes a valid consent to screening and whether screening is ever lawful without express consent. The difficulties inherent in understanding the common law are exacerbated by the fact that even within the common law there is no discrete body of principles exclusively relevant to health care law. Principles defining patients' rights and professional obligations have to be deduced from generally applicable rules of criminal law and tort. The legality of screening for HIV largely concerns the laws relating to the crime of assault, and the torts of trespass to the person and negligence. It should be noted that in the absence of legislation or express legal precedents on screening, the courts are likely to give great weight to the considered opinion of the professional regulatory bodies, in particular the General Medical Council (GMC) and the United Kingdom Central Council for Nurses, Midwives and Health Visitors (UKCC).

The ethicist is concerned to identify how individuals should relate to each other and to the society in which they live. Thus, ethicists are primarily concerned to develop models of ethical behaviour — ideals. The lawyer then has to ask three questions:

1. Is there a consensus on a particular model of ethical behaviour?

2. If there is, by what practical means can the rights and obligations consequent on that model be enforced?

3. To what extent in the enforcement process, do we want or need to use some sort of coercive sanctions to forward that process?

In many areas of health care and bioethics, the first question about consensus on an appropriate model of ethical behaviour is more or less irresoluble. If we were addressing the advances in embryology or the application of genetics, consensus would be an absolute miracle, the like of which has not been seen for 2,000 years.

Fortunately, in the context of screening for HIV, I think there is more or less a consensus on the proper model of ethical behaviour. There must be — to put it at its lowest — the strongest presumption that when testing poses such awesome implications for the individual herself, for her future and for her family, every individual who is to be tested has the right to make a truly autonomous and informed judgement whether or not to undergo testing. That right may not necessarily be absolute — Professor Harris has suggested that it is not — but any derogation from that right requires the strictest justification.

There is, as far as I can see, little or no support for any universal policy of mandatory or compulsory testing. There is universal condemnation of any sort of practice of surreptitious testing, where the subject gives consent to the taking of blood but is denied proper information about the purpose or implications of what is to be done, whether it is testing for HIV or testing to identify some genetic disorder.

If there is some agreement on the model of behaviour, how does English law enforce that model? Parliament has elected to leave these issues largely to the common law. The only relevant legislation is the HIV Testing Kits and Services Regulations 1992 made under the Health and Medicines Act 1988 to prevent unauthorized persons marketing or using HIV testing kits. Screening is to be entrusted to the medical profession. The judgement of medical professionals, subject to their own ethical codes of practice and ultimately to the courts, is presumably considered sufficient to achieve the proper aim of screening. But how effective are the ultimate judicial controls? In England they depend on general principles governing consent to treatment, which, in turn, derive from age-old rules originally designed simply to control physical violence. Any physical contact with another person, however slight, constitutes the crime of assault and the tort of trespass, unless expressly or implicitly authorized by the person touched.

Here is the first problem which Professor Harris identifies: the rules relating to assault which protect an individual's bodily integrity operate only if there is some touching — for example, the use of a needle to take blood from an arm. Consider for the moment the use of blood for screening. Any doctor taking blood from me for screening purposes must have my consent. Blood is often taken from a patient for a host of purposes. How much must the doctor tell the patient about the tests which he proposes to conduct on her blood? The agreed ethical model is that if it is proposed to screen blood for HIV or to test for genetic disorder, the subject must be told exactly what is envisaged and should receive adequate, preferably independent, counselling on the implications of agreeing to the relevant tests. If crucial information is withheld on the purpose of testing and its implications, does this make the apparent consent invalid? Does it expose the doctor to liability for assault? An English judge ruled in a different context that a failure to explain the risks and implications of [proposed] treatment does not invalidate consent. For a consent to be valid, all the patient need be told is: "in broad terms of the nature of the procedure which is intended" (Chatterton v Gerson [1981] 1 All ER 257).

So in normal circumstances, a failure to canvass with the patient the implications of agreeing to treatment does not invalidate consent.

What exactly is meant in English law by the "nature of the procedure"? What is the nature of the procedure if blood is taken for testing purposes? At one level, it is simply: "I would like to stick a needle in your arm and draw out blood." Patients who are scheduled for surgery have blood taken for a variety of reasons. They are asked for consent to testing prior to surgery, to cross-match blood and to test for a host of possible conditions. They are not told exactly what tests will be performed.

In relation to HIV, however, we say that the patient must be expressly informed if, among that battery of tests which it is intended to carry out, is an HIV test. There is great disagreement among lawyers in England about whether a failure to tell a patient that the doctor plans to test for HIV would render what is being done to the patient an assault. The lawyers advising the British Medical Association (BMA) argue cogently that a diagnosis of HIV has such profound implications for, and can cause such damage to the patient that a test for HIV is quite different in nature from all the other usual categories of tests.

The difficulty with the argument is that it has not been common in the United Kingdom to give patients specific information on the type and purposes of diagnostic tests. Pregnant women are routinely tested for syphilis. Few are ever told that on occasion the blood taken will be tested for syphilis. Most women presumably assume, as I did, that blood is being taken simply for the usual purposes of checking on their general health and to screen for all the various conditions which can develop in pregnancy, such as anaemia and diabetes.

A large number of antenatal clinics still do not tell the woman when blood is being taken to test for raised levels of alpha-protein. The first she knows about it is when, if she does have a raised level of alpha-protein, she receives a letter asking her to attend the clinic to consider far more intensive and invasive antenatal screening.

Patients are being tested for conditions they are not told about every day. Is HIV so different in nature from all other diseases that it is clear beyond doubt that withholding information of the intent to test for HIV invalidates consent altogether? Alternatively, are obstetricians in the United Kingdom routinely assaulting pregnant patients when testing for syphilis or checking alpha-protein levels?

However, the law does not simply concern itself with the question of assault. The judge who set that very minimal threshold for an effective consent, who said that for consent to be effective there is no need to canvass the implications of treatment, went on to say that nonetheless there is a duty of care to provide careful counselling on the risks and implications of treatment. A doctor failing to provide adequate information and advice to assist the patient to decide whether or not to agree to a particular treatment or test, might not be liable for assault, but he could be liable for negligence.

If the law does require that relevant information be provided for a patient, it might be asked why lawyers waste so much energy disputing whether or not consent is invalidated, and whether there is an assault. If there is an obligation which the law will ultimately enforce, is not that enough?

English judges have been assiduous in their attempts to protect medical professionals from criminal responsibility in the context of their obligations to patients generally, and in particular in relation to matters of consent to treatment. Patient autonomy is thought to be sufficiently protected by the civil — the non-criminal — rules governing relations between individuals. Monetary compensation is deemed a sufficient remedy for all but the most outrageous violations of patient autonomy.

Whether this is correct requires us to ask:

1. How useful are civil remedies if there is no money to pursue them?

2. Is it right to say that something as fundamental as the right to autonomy, to self determination, is a purely personal interest, in the enforcement of which society as a whole has no particular role?

3. Is the civil remedy in negligence adequate?

The last question is perhaps the most important. The courts have said that it is part of the doctor's duty to give her patients adequate information, but who defines the standard, the content, of that information? What does "informed consent" entail in England? The shortanswer is "not much".

In the famous case of Sidaway v Royal Bethlem Hospital ([1985] 1 All ER 643) and a series of subsequent judgements, the Law Lords and the Court of Appeal have consistently ruled that the amount of information and advice to which English patients are entitled is governed by the professional standard. Provided that a medical practitioner provides his patients with that degree of information and advice considered appropriate by a responsible body of professional opinion, he has discharged his legal obligation. In effect, this means that provided that the medical practitioner whose patient believes her autonomy has been violated can find three or four sufficiently distinguished experts to say "I would have done just as Dr Bloggs did", any civil remedy is unlikely to succeed. As long as the doctor gives the patient as much information as fellow professionals would consider necessary, he is not negligent. The House of Lords has expressly rejected the view now endorsed by the Supreme Courts of Canada and Australia that the standard should be based on the information which a reasonable, prudent patient would desire in order to make an informed choice.

Now it might be asked whether this matters in the context of HIV. In the context of screening for HIV and genetic disorder, distinguished medical practitioners agree that their patients are entitled to adequate information and counselling. It is clear that the health care professions themselves, through formal advice from regulatory bodies such as the GMC, opinions expressed by the BMA, and the overwhelming weight of opinion expressed by leading HIV specialists, accept that as a general rule a health professional must (1) always disclose any intent to test for HIV and (2) fully advise and counsel the patient on the consequences of agreeing to screening. Both the psychological consequences of a positive result and the potential adverse consequences on financial and insurance status of agreeing to testing at all, must be fully canvassed with the patient. The professional standard perhaps enforces a patient's right to information sufficiently to protect that patient against any maverick member of the profession? In theory, perhaps, but in practice I have some doubts. The Royal College of Surgeons (RCS) has issued guidelines authorizing non-consensual testing in exceptional circumstances. If an accident occurs, risking blood-to-blood contact between patient and surgeon, and if there is some reason to believe that the patient might be HIV-positive, I understand that the RCS guidelines provide that the surgeon may test the patient's blood there and then, without waiting to obtain any express consent.

So there is a responsible body of opinion endorsing, albeit only in exceptional circumstances, involuntary testing. More worryingly though, than this exceptional case, conversations with surgeons lead me to believe that a number of them would like to go rather further, and would like to see much more widespread pre-operative HIV testing. Their argument is that they routinely test for every other "nasty" without explaining very much to the patient, so why do they not test for what might be described as the most dangerous "nasty"?

Far more widespread non-consensual testing takes place in the United Kingdom within the scheme for monitoring the spread of HIV. Blood taken for other purposes in, amongst other places, antenatal clinics and certain general practitioner (GP) clinics, is sent, with all identifying factors removed from the sample, for HIV testing. If the BMA is right, and testing my blood for HIV without my express consent is a criminal assault, why are such practices not assaults? One official argument goes as follows: leaflets and notices prepared by the Department of Health are available in National Health Service clinics, explaining to patients that after their blood has been tested for the purposes they have agreed, some residual blood may be forwarded for unlinked anonymised HIV testing. The patient is invited to inform the doctor, or whoever else is taking blood, if she objects. If she says nothing, consent is to be presumed.

Apart from the fact that those leaflets are more often absent than present, the problem with this argument is that passive consent is a notion entirely alien to English law. Let us assume that I write to Lord Kennet offering to buy his London house for £20,000. I say to him that, if I hear nothing from him before 31 January, I shall presume that he consents. On 1 February, I take my Pickford's van there to move in. Nobody would suggest that Lord Kennet is now bound to hand over to me his London residence.

Perhaps, in focusing so narrowly on the question of consent, we miss the point. The RCS permits exceptional non-consensual testing because of evidence — disputed I know, but evidence with which the RCS is satisfied — that immediate prophylactic therapy may reduce the risk of infection to an individual exposed to HIV. The RCS argument would be that a surgeon who has been exposed to a potentially lethal risk is entitled to act in self defence. In relation to epidemiological screening for HIV, Professor Harris has said that it is designed to enable those responsible for public health to devise the best possible strategy to limit the spread of disease: the Department of Health acts in defence of the community. The crux of the issue is not so much whether there has been a violation of autonomy — because I think undoubtedly there has been — but whether this is one of the exceptional circumstances where that violation is justifiable.

The current legal mechanisms controlling screening for disease make no allowance for this factor, save when statute has prescribed that the public health interest outweighs the private right. So the Public Health (Control of Disease) Act 1984, and the Regulations made under it, enable community health officers to require individuals to be tested for certain diseases. If there was any suspicion that the stomach upset which affected me last night was cholera, it would be perfectly permissible for doctors to have me tested immediately, regardless of whether or not I agreed to such a test. But HIV is not one of those diseases for which statute provides for any form of non-consensual testing — albeit, ironically, a patient with acquired immune deficiency syndrome (full blown AIDS) can in some circumstances be compulsorily detained for treatment under that Act on the order of a magistrate.

No allowance is made in the common law rules for the "public interest", in sharp contrast to the complementary rules governing medical confidentiality. The absolutist nature of the consent rules is perhaps in part responsible for the rather arid and limited interpretation of those rules by English judges. They are worried about bringing the blunderbuss of the criminal law into play to correct what is seen as a flawed doctor-patient relationship.

In looking for the sorts of mechanisms which might better regulate the doctor-patient relationship, in the general context, as well as in the specific context of screening, in Canada there is a new dawn breaking. The Supreme Court of Canada is a unique institution which draws its judges both from the English-speaking common law tradition and from the French-speaking civil law tradition of Quebec. They have been forced — as the European Union is being forced — to find some way of marrying the common and civil law traditions.

The Canadian Supreme Court has now categorized the doctor-patient relationship as a fiduciary relationship akin to that of parent and child, or guardian and ward, or trustee and beneficiary. It has said that the fundamental obligation of the doctor is to act with the utmost good faith and loyalty. The implications of this relationship remain to be worked out, and indeed there are disagreements on how to proceed within the Canadian Supreme Court itself.

One particular judgement of the Supreme Court shows the capacity of this legal mechanism, the fiduciary relationship, to get around the difficulties of rules which rest on assault and battery. In a case, Norberg v Wynrib ([1992] 92 DLR 449), an elderly doctor had supplied drugs to an addicted female patient on condition that she accorded him sexual favours. In her action against the doctor for the considerable harm which ensued to her, three of the judges struggled with the thorny topic of whether her "apparent" consent was real or overborne by coercion. Mrs Justice McLachlin and one of her colleagues from

Quebec said quite openly that they regarded the issue of whether or not there had been an assault and whether there was a real consent as something of a red herring. There could be no doubt that the core of the doctor's misbehaviour was his abuse of the trust of the patient. If you focus on the decision of Ms Norberg to submit to Dr Wynrib and say, as Mrs Justice McLachlin's colleagues did, that there was no real consent there, that she was probably not competent to consent, that she was coerced, then question marks are raised about the competence of addicted patients to consent to all sorts of other things. A possible consequence of such an argument is that the autonomy of the others is undermined for the purpose of achieving what everybody agreed was the right result for Ms Norberg.

Mrs Justice McLachlin said: "An unjustified abuse of power within a fiduciary relationship must be unlawful." She freed herself to look at the particular needs of that particular patient. She enabled herself to treat consent and confidentiality, not as two separate and isolated legal questions, but very much one and the same. A satisfactory means of ensuring confidentiality, as Professor Harris has said, is in many circumstances the best means of obtaining a truly voluntary and informed consent to treatment.

Whether the English courts will be prepared to accept and extend a notion of a fiduciary relationship, more commonly thought of in the context of property — entrusting our money to the bank and our mortgage to the solicitor — than in the context of personal relations is unclear at present. However, I think that any difficulties can be overcome, by legislation if necessary.

We need to find a way in which the law can effectively ensure that information disclosure and the consent process in screening, both for HIV and for genetic disorder, meet the actual and real needs of the particular patient in the particular context in which screening is proposed. Any derogation from the duty of utmost good faith and protection of the patient's interests should be justifiable only in the most exceptional circumstances where the interests of others must manifestly take priority over the interests of the patient. In the context of screening both for HIV and for genetic disorder, it may well be that only Parliaments by legislation should take on that role, and not leave such judgments either to individual medical professionals or to individual judges.

Let me end more or less where I began. Does the law matter? There is no concrete evidence of wholesale coercion of patients. Does this show that the current legal rules are perhaps good enough? I beg to differ. The key word is evidence. There is little empirical evidence about what is actually going on. All we know is that there have not been any lawsuits as yet. The lack of a clear and coherent legal basis for screening has led to a degree of confusion about the state of the law among health care professionals, and to a scheme for monitoring the spread of HIV, the legality of which is dubious, to say the least.

*
* *

Discussion*

Discussion focused on three broad topics: (1) counselling and information provision; (2) access to insurance and to medical resources; and (3) moral issues raised by the competing demands of autonomy and privacy, on the one hand, and (what one might label) civic responsibility, on the other. A further category, (4) miscellaneous remarks, is introduced to capture submissions of interest which fall outside the first three

---

* Professor D. Giesen (Dean of Law, Free University of Berlin, Germany) substituted for Professor Brazier in this discussion.

categories. Needless to say, the categories overlap to some extent.

Counselling and information provision

Sherr: First, I endorse the claim made by Professor Harris, that counselling should be objective, but much of the practice, especially with HIV, is to train the primary worker to do the counselling. If the primary person who is taking the blood, is doing the counselling, can she be objective? Secondly, about the provision of information within counselling. Perhaps we should ask whether we are really saying that people need accurate information prior to making a decision. This might change the economic basis of providing such counselling, and might preserve genuine counselling for those who need it.

Harris: I failed to distinguish between those two sorts of counselling. I was putting together the information-giving and the facilitation of decision-making dimensions of counselling. They should be separated.

The question of objectivity is complicated: it is not whether someone can be completely objective, but whether an attempt is being made. Some constraints will be financial: can we afford to separate the counsellors? Can some societies afford even to provide counselling? When we use a term like "objective", we have to qualify it by saying "as objective as possible" within a range of constraints, some of which will be changeable, and some of which will not.

Austin: In Italy, counselling is currently provided by medical care-givers who have no training in providing basic counselling. I am aware of a number of community-based organizations in developing countries that provide excellent counselling skills. The concept of adequate counselling is part of the problem here: can counselling be provided only by professionally trained, qualified personnel — for example, someone who has a degree in psychology or in medicine?

Giesen: Counselling must be as objective as possible, but who will define what is objective? Are we leaving it to the professionals, whatever the profession — the medics perhaps, as the Bolam-test in this country would imply? This is not heard of in any other legal system.

As long as screening discovers deficiencies in individuals, be it only the wrong sex, if we cannot offer alternatives, or if the only alternative is killing (think of India or other places when a child of the wrong sex is born), or if deficiencies are discovered like HIV and AIDS which are not treatable, whom does the screening help and who are the victims when there is no available therapy?

Harris: What should our response be to things to which we do not yet have an answer? Should we halt things while lawyers, philosophers and theologians look for answer? As I am sure Dr Giesen recognizes, this would be practically impossible, and I am not even sure that it would be theoretically desirable. It is not the research that should be halted, or have a moratorium put on it, but, as with the information, its use for particular problems should not be allowed until the questions have been resolved.

Nairne: Would Professor Harris see an ethical imperative to provide relevant and good sex education in schools? It is a matter that goes wider than teaching about sex. We are talking about teaching about human relations. How, in particular, should the question of homosexuality — very relevant to HIV and AIDS — be dealt with?

Harris: Briefly, it is imperative that AIDS education starts early, and starts in schools. In the United Kingdom, we are reasonably well placed to carry public opinion with us on this, but there are many communities, not only within Europe but outside it, where this would be impossible. At a recent AIDS conference in Japan, it was made clear that, in Japan, it would be unacceptable to have sex education in schools, let alone education about homosexuality, promiscuity and so on.

I am less clear how we should educate about homosexuality. It depends on whether there is any reliable information that homosexuality is a more risky sexuality than heterosexuality. It seems unlikely that it is not *in toto*, as it were, for historical rather than intrinsic reasons. My own view is that homosexuality should be treated exactly like heterosexuality, both for the age of consent, and for the views we take about the desirability of people indulging in it. I do not see that it would need to be made part of an AIDS education programme in schools, although I think it would be desirable to include it.

Marteau: Few of us would disagree that education or counselling is a good thing, but where is the evidence that it makes any difference? It is unethical to spend money on counselling if we do not know whether it will have any effect. This is a plea for some evidence.

Harris: Whether there is any evidence that education, for example, makes a difference depends on what difference we are looking for. If it is an increase in autonomy — *i.e.* the ability to make a rational choice if you wish to — it clearly does make a difference. If it is reduction of AIDS-incidence, there is no evidence that the two are connected. It may be important to have an increase in autonomy even if the number of people who contract AIDS is not thereby reduced. People cannot be made to accept advice, but they can be given the advice they need to decide whether or not they wish to run a risk.

Marteau: I want to know what you mean by autonomy. As Sir Patrick Nairne suggested, the issue is not just about the biology of sex, but about human relationships. I would still argue that some evidence is needed that education might increase people's autonomy, enabling them to decide whether or not to use a condom.

Harris: I agree in principle. I agree that knowing you are at large risk if you have unprotected sexual intercourse in a context in which you do not feel able to insist upon protected intercourse may be worth less to you than if both partners have the autonomy that knowledge provides, and the necessary power along with it.

Super: Counselling can be directive or non-directive. Where both AIDS and genetic disorders are concerned, I do not think education or the counselling process can be purely non-directive, nor do I feel that we need to have a conscience about it. Society is entitled to try to direct people towards how bad some of these things are, to allow them free choice but also to help them make what we hope would be sensible decisions. I think it is quite reasonable to look at incidences of AIDS to see how successful counselling issues are.

Austin: Evidence is available that education lowers the incidence of HIV-infection. In Denmark there has been sex education in schools for 20-30 years, whereas in Italy there is still no formal sex education. There have been attempts to introduce literature discussing AIDS in the Italian school system, but the literature was banned because it discussed condom use. Currently the average age of a diagnosed AIDS case in Italy is 25-30 years old, which means that these people are probably being infected during adolescence. There are 18,000 young people diagnosed with AIDS in Italy, and at least 100,000 people infected. This is largely because there is no sex education.

Exon: Who has recently published a paper showing that sexual health education given to young people (I avoid saying in schools) delays sexual debut rather than encourages them to experiment.

Partridge: I am surprised, and saddened, that education programmes were so quickly questioned today. A number of surveys have clearly shown that early sex education results in starting sex later, lowered rates of unwanted teenage pregnancy, and increased condom use. Given that, with HIV, there are both the costs of long-term care amongst young people and the additional costs of lost economic input into a society, I think the cost-benefit of education strategies are absolutely clear.

The issue of counselling is more difficult. The most effective counselling settings — both pre- and post-test — are where there is the greatest input, which costs the most. I think we have an ethical dilemma of whether to invest in the high cost of long-term counselling or just to ignore counselling altogether.

Access to insurance and medical resources

Holm: Professor Harris ended his presentation by saying that insurers should have no access to any health information. Would he extend that outside the health care sector? Let us say that I have a house that is burning, although at the moment very slowly, and I approach him for insurance against fire. Would that not be a parallel to the patient who is HIV-positive and would now like to take out a life insurance policy?

Harris: It is a parallel, but not an exact one. It is a complicated issue. We would have to take steps against deliberate fraud. If we were to move to a system in which insurance was provided on the basis of statistical information only, rather than on the basis of individual information, it might well be that limits would be set on the sort of insurance that could be obtained under that rubric, so that people would not be able to "clean up" on the basis of a known risk. The system might also have to be subsidized in some way.

Because the ability to obtain insurance cover is linked in many societies with the capacity to obtain medical treatment, and in others (*e.g.* the United Kingdom) with the capacity to own houses, my point was that it is essential to have some way of providing insurance in a context in which increasingly reliable information will be easily and generally available via human genome analysis, genetic screening and so on. It will be as essential for the survival of the insurance industry as for the survival of civil liberties and equality.

Van Damme: Insurance companies should not have the right to do any testing. In Western European countries, we live in a society with a tradition of social security systems. If private insurance companies are allowed to test, they will be able to offer much cheaper insurance than that offered through social security systems. This might lead to dividing society into those who have all the advantages and those who haven't. It would make the cost both for health care and insurance much higher for those who need it most. This is the political choice that has to be made.

Kennet: Professor Harris called for a kind of health insurance which would not ask for any individual health particulars, and would simply look at the person to see his/her sex and age. This would require a fairly massive reform of what happens now. They have asked for health details over many decades.

Giesen: I am sceptical that we can avoid insurance companies having access to the information which is available by one means or another. I have my doubts whether ethicists, philosophers and lawyers together will ever solve this problem. There is already so much information on our credit cards, health insurance policy schemes, etc. I think all the information which can be gathered will be used, sometimes by the right people, sometimes by the wrong ones; and competition will ensure that the insurance companies do not run too great a risk with individuals whom they want to avoid including in their insurance schemes. This applies to all the minorities mentioned by Professor Harris, including the smokers.

Harris: I agree that where there is information, people will obtain it. Therefore, our only hope is not to control access to information but to control its use. The extent to which we are entitled in a free society to control the use of information is a political as well as an ethical question. I was impressed by Dr van Damme's comment that if insurance companies are allowed to "clean up" on those who present virtually no risk, leaving the state or society to pick up the bill for the rest, many societies would regard that not as in the public interest — even societies that would generally defend a free market.

Large: I am the Managing Director of BUPA, the principal health insurance company in the United Kingdom. First, all of us in business operate within the ethical framework set by the bodies that this conference is seeking to influence and also within the ethical view of public opinion. Insurance companies do not use all the data at their disposal to distinguish various risks. If we did, most young males would be charged more than young females, and vice versa in later years of life. This is not done because it is not acceptable to public opinion. (Smoking and obesity are becoming issues, an appeal to which in risk-assessment is acceptable to public opinion.)

As to seeking to prohibit health insurance companies from any testing, the essential difference between health insurance and other forms of insurance is that the individual has a far greater knowledge about his likely risk than anybody else, other than his general practitioner, could possibly obtain. He is therefore in a position to bias strongly the risk-relationship with the insurer. This is why life insurance, until the last couple of decades, has excluded suicide as a reason for reimbursement. People with serious illness are in a not dissimilar circumstance.

Would the state end up supporting all those who could not afford the insurance premium for their risk? The question arises when we start to use insurance to cover large parts of the population (in Germany, for instance).

Harris: I am pleased to hear Mr Large defend the principle of regulation, and effectively say that it is in the self interest of the British insurance industry to stay a small part of the market. I would be interested to see whether that is reflected in its advertising.

Sandberg: Professor Harris' policy proposals for insurance are quite radical. In Europe there are two kinds of insurance systems that seem to work:

— public health insurance, which is compulsory and community-rated, for which individuals pay according to their income, not according to their risk;
— private risk-rated insurance which is fully voluntary — except in Britain, I think, where there is this rule of mortgage and house owning which complicates the system.

Instead of stopping insurers asking about risk-information in the private market, it might be better to move everything that it is considered people really need into the community-rated market.

I think Professor Harris' last suggestion about the sort of limited community-rated insurance with a questioning limit is worth considering further, for I know that it is working in the Netherlands. What would it cost, and how feasible is it? I have calculated the cost for Norway, where we are fortunate to have only a very few people with HIV (1,200-1,300 in a population of four millions). Suppose a questioning limit were introduced, and put at twice the average individual life insurance size today, and insurers were not allowed to ask about HIV below this level. If everyone with HIV bought life insurance (which probably they would not) and they all died within ten years (these are very pessimistic assumptions), the premium increase on average would be £2.70 per person, a 1.5% increase, which seems quite small.

Draper: Two questions that need to be answered are:

1. Do insurance companies need to provide insurance?
2. Are insurance companies obliged to provide insurance?

Insurance companies do not need to provide insurance. People talk as though insurance companies would just carry on trading at a deficit. They would not; they would just stop trading. They need to make money. And insurance companies are not obliged to provide insurance at a loss to themselves. If we tell insurance companies that they cannot leave people at high risk without health care, we have to ask what obligation that places on us. The insurance companies can be obliged to insure everybody only if everyone is equally obliged to buy insurance.

De Wachter: The Dutch system, very much like the one that was just described, is a two-tier-system of health insurance. The life insurers have made a gentlemen's agreement with the Dutch Government whereby, for five years from 1989, they abstained from asking questions about either genetic information or the HIV serostatus of people, and from doing additional testing, provided that the insurance cover was less than 200,000 guilders (about $40,000).

Too little time has passed to evaluate what has been done. Part of the agreement was that after five years they would report to the government on the outcome. There are two major problems with the outcome: (1) the life insurers do not know — and they believe it is not possible to find out — how many people have abstained from applying for life insurance; (2) it is impossible to know how many people applied but did not give information about HIV or genetic disease.

Why do we talk about no information or a little information? Why not talk about all the information? A policy study in the Netherlands has tried to explain that it might work from the viewpoint of social justice if it were compulsory to give all medical information (and therefore all genetic and HIV information) to the life insurers. Of course, the first real result would be that individuals would become victims: they will be ostracized and so on, as has been rightly said. But what if society were to set up a system whereby the individual, or his or her family, were not the victims, instead creating the funds by tax deduction, to compensate for the rise in premium which those people would have to pay? This would have the advantage that we would work with full knowledge instead of limited knowledge as at present. We could monitor developments, and not play a game, with one individual lucky and another unlucky.

Harris: I was interested in Dr de Wachter's suggestion. Assuming that both suggestions would solve the problem (which may be an assumption many people would not accept), namely, the problem of providing health care and protection for all the people in the community, the only difference between them is whether it is desirable on other grounds for hugely important personal information about any individual to be generally known or not.

I can think of many reasons why people would wish to confine information — for example, relatively reliable information about the lifespan of an individual which may be provided by genetic screening. Are they likely to die in mid-life rather than in old age? Many people would be uncomfortable about this information being generally known if there were no practical reason why it should be generally known. They would feel uncomfortable even if it was not likely to be used against them in all sorts of other ways, not just in the provision of insurance but in employment and in their social acceptability. It has to be recognized that not only employment and insurance, but views about the right to reproduce and the rights to a range of other things in society, are likely to be influenced, I think wrongly, by knowledge about people's health status and life expectancy.

Pembrey: From the insurance point of view, in a situation in which the genotype determines whether an individual gets a disease — *i.e.* if the genotype is present, he will get the disease, and if it is not, he will not develop it: for example, something like Huntington's chorea — it is true to say that the genotype is equivalent to a specific risk for a specific disease. But these simply inherited disorders are relatively rare and do not constitute any real financial threat to the insurance company in terms of bias.

Dixon: On the question of self destructive behaviour, I wholeheartedly agree with Professor Harris' argument that we should not seek to divide AIDS victims into innocent and guilty categories. On a broader front, however, he was very much opposed to the notion, which is gaining ground in various places, that people who indulge in self destructive behaviour should have a lesser priority in terms of access to medical resources. I am thinking here of the smoker with cardiovascular problems, the alcoholic with cirrhosis who wants a liver transplant, and so forth.

How far can the argument be pressed that these considerations should never have any weight? Clearly, they will be exacerbated by genetic screening; for example, in each of the two cases I have mentioned, there may well be predisposing genes. Do we say that those considerations should never be weighed, or perhaps that people who indulge in self destructive behaviour of that sort are so few that we can afford to ignore the problem?

Harris: My main plea is for consistency. One consistent approach — although not one that I would favour — is if we are prepared to say that everybody who is in any degree responsible for his adverse health state should either get no care or have low priority. It would have to be applied consistently across society. Thus, if you volunteer to be a policeman, you are increasing your risk of being a victim of assault by criminals, so a policeman who is a victim of such an assault is responsible for the adverse health state that is a consequence. As it happens, by and large, we approve of people being policemen, so we tend to exempt them. The same is true of sportsmen and a range of other activities.

I am implacably opposed to the way we disguise our moral prejudices about certain habits, lifestyles or social practices as a concern for justice or impartiality in the degree of health care. It is nothing of the sort. If we are prepared to be consistent, we have to look at all occupational risks, sports, a range of diets, a predilection for other forms of food that have been shown to have adverse health risks and so on, but which are not yet as unacceptable as smoking and alcoholism. When we see the extent to which almost all of us are implicated in adverse health risks to some extent, the whole thing becomes unworkable.

Autonomy, privacy, and civic responsibility

Young: How will all these things fit into a general idea of a social contract, which is, to some extent, what we are talking about? The social contract — roughly, between each citizen and all citizens including each citizen — is an organic mixture of rights and duties which change as time passes. What are the rights and duties of the community towards the individual in this field? There has been a lot of emphasis on autonomy, but what are the duties of the individual towards the community?

The Chinese Government, which is now proposing eugenic regulations, says that there are at least ten million Chinese alive whose births could usefully have been prevented. The USA immigration services have attempted to keep out of the USA people who are HIV seropositive. Both the Chinese and the American governments were considering the rights of the community at large to be more important than the autonomy of individuals.

Giesen: It is right to question the notion of autonomy if it is not complemented by a notion of responsibility. With regard to the social contract between individuals and society, we may ask the simple question whether individuals have any right to health care. This is not such a silly question as it sounds. We are the happy Europeans here. In the American scenario, 40 million citizens are not insured at all, or are underinsured, so there is this basic question of whether we have a right to health care. If weanswer in the affirmative (which we should be quick in doing), the second question is how much health care we have a right to. Is there a right merely to basic treatment, or to all sorts of heroic treatment, such as artificial reproduction, having babies at 59 or 60, and cost-intensive high-tech procedures? If there is such a right it will rob our society of money which even in the First World is needed for basic treatment.

This is a sinister question, but I think society can demand, at least to some extent, that certain minorities, such as smokers, behave more reasonably.

Bennedsen: Compulsory testing has been discussed in the Danish Parliament and, except for the one really right-wing party, there was agreement that we should not have it. The reason was primarily that we believe a policy based on open information, the voluntary principle and anonymity is the best way to combat HIV-infection. Furthermore, the result of the test is not useful because it provides knowledge of the HIV status 3-6 months ago, not the current status; such a test would have to be done every three months, and that would be very expensive.

There is an ethical problem with testing which has not been mentioned. I understand there are 5% — 10% false positives. To make testing compulsory, thereby putting 5% or 10% of people in that situation, raises an ethical problem.

Serfaty: The principles of HIV testing policy in France are based on voluntarism and self-responsibility for safe health behaviour. In 1988 the Ministry of Health implemented free and anonymous HIV testing and couselling sites: there are more than 180 sites throughout France, implemented either in STD clinics or in hospitals. The health professionals working in these centres are trained for pre- and post-test counselling.

For three years there has been great controversy over mandatory HIV testing. Two amendments were proposed by the Senate in the Autumn of 1993, namely:

— mandatory HIV testing for patients with tuberculosis;
— systematically proposed, HIV testing for prisoners.

Arguments were then presented that these legislative instruments were unnecessary given existing medical practice. They have now been cancelled by Parliament, and we shall be debating testing policies in the spring (1994).

Serrao: Do you think that, in the near future, screening for HIV and AIDS will, or will not, be obligatory? My point is that if there is not the possibility of a treatment soon, screening will be obligatory by public demand.

Harris: The answer is simple: even if it were desirable, the cost would make it not in the public interest on economic grounds alone, given the expected level of risk. It is expensive to test an entire population.

Serrao: It will become cheaper soon.

Harris: The next thing we would need to know is in what sense testing the entire population would protect anybody. It might protect the insurance companies, but it would not diminish the level of risk of contracting HIV in the community.

Giesen: If the right to self-determination, alluded to by Professor Harris and Professor Brazier, means the right to know everything, the flip-side of the coin is the right not to know about one's status. Should society know more than I want to know myself?

Iglesias: In talking about the reciprocity of obligations. I think that we cannot take "society" as a moral or legal person to whom we have obligations. Can Dr Giesen or any other lawyer say whether it is true that society is never as such a legal person, that legal obligations are always between individuals? Professor Brazier mentioned the guidelines of the Royal College of Surgeons in England. If there is an accident, and an injured person is bleeding, for the safety of the surgeons themselves it is compulsory to test that person for HIV or any other condition. This is understandable because there is a reciprocal obligation there: on the part of the patient the obligation is not to harm, on the part of the surgeons (medical staff) the right not to be harmed.

Giesen: I would have no disagreement with Professor Brazier in answering the question about whether society could be treated as a legal person. The basic answer that lawyers would give is that we are all individuals, we are the ones who have rights. Society as such does not have legal personality; rather the state, constituted by law, is the relevant legal person. Thus, the state may be subjected to legal obligations towards its citizens, for example under the rule of *habeas corpus*, and may subject itself to obligations to other states, for example by way of international treaties. The term "society", therefore, is best confined to the pre-legal discourse of philosophy and sociology. The interests of society in public health and the control of disease are advanced by the state through enacted and, in Common Law countries, judge-made law. The powers of the state to advance these interests are, however, limited by the rights of individual citizens. Thus, the right of liberty or individual autonomy may limit, or "trump" the power of state authorities to implement compulsory testing for HIV. For health boards or hospitals, to test a patient's blood for HIV antibodies without his consent or without other legal justification (*e.g.* contagious diseases legislation) would constitute a grave violation of that person's fundamental right to self-determination, leaving the parties involved open to both civil and criminal liability. In fact most western countries do not impose an obligation upon individuals to undergo such tests. That said, an individual may be subject to a duty at civil law to make disclosure of his HIV positive status, if this is necessary to avert a serious and real threat to the health of others, including, in this context, health care professionals.

Miscellaneous

Wehkamp: A broad range of information is needed to give good therapy in AIDS. The special nature of the disease is that it is an illness of the biological self defence system, and will thus potentially be an aspect of any other illness or injury that has to be treated in affected individuals. This must be considered in talking about screening in the context of medical treatment, and I have missed this today.

There could be a conflict between the principles of autonomy and the duty of a surgeon to know the complete medical status of a patient, and to provide a therapy orientated to the whole person and his whole biological system. I do not think that good medicine can be given without information on the immunological status of a person.

Pembrey: Consider the angiotensin-converting enzyme. The population is divided into two groups, about half of whom have a different variant of this gene from the others. The so-called "deletion" variant was shown to increase an individual's risk of myocardial infarct. A study was done, and this variant was labelled as a 2 "at-risk" genotype for myocardial infarct — clearly something that the insurance companies would like to look at. A study of centenarians, just published from France, has shown, much to everybody's surprise, that they had a greater percentage of individuals with this "at-risk" genotype!

We run into real trouble if we start medicalizing genetic variation. If that is avoided, we are talking about relatively small numbers — something that the insurance companies, the public and the interested genetic lay groups can sort out.

Harris: I am interested in what you say, but surely your objection was not to the medicalization of the information but only to its unreliability. You were implying that it would be all right if reliable statistical judgements could be made about people's life expectancy with particular genotypes. What would you say if we were able to make reliable estimates about, for example, people's life expectancy or susceptibility to heart disease with particular genotypes?

Pembrey: I beg to differ, although of course we might like to have reliable predictions. Take a genetic variation we can all see, blond hair and fair skin. We do not refer to those people as being "at-risk" of sunburn, although they are. Indeed, their sensitivity to the sun is probably helpful in advising everybody that the sun is dangerous, that we should protect the ozone layer and so on. It is genuinely a question of attitude. If we want to get increasing amounts of information from the genotype instead of from the environment, we will run into trouble.

A final point is that the new techniques in genetic testing analysis are so powerful that very small genotypic differences between groups can be detected. It is paradoxical that the genetic differences between two groups are revealed when the total population is put under environmental stress. Initially, the more the environmental stress, the more the genetic differences will be revealed between those who succumb and those who can cope. Eventually, environmental stress overwhelms all genotypes. So, paradoxically, when genetic differences are found it may indicate that there are environmental stresses that ought to be looked at and dealt with, not that the individuals should be labelled as "ill" because of their genetic variation.

Harris: You are saying that when there are rival therapies for the same problem, there may be political and moral reasons to prefer one of them. If the only problem single parents have is the prejudice of society, two actions are possible: to eradicate single parents or to try to eradicate the prejudice. I agree that it is better to work on the latter.

In the case of genetic predisposition to, say, environmental vulnerability, such as being blond and pale skinned and susceptibility to melanoma, if it is possible to work on the environment, that is what should be done. However there may be situations where this cannot be done, and if it is possible to work on the genome to afford protection which no other policy can afford, it seems to me that we should not turn our backs on that alternative by pretending that operating on the genome is not a form of treating the problem.

Pembrey: I was not really getting into the question of operating on the genome — that is presumably gene therapy. Where there is a genetic defect which causes a devastating disease and which can be dealt with by gene therapy, that is not different from other types of therapy. The issue is not that, but that the insurance companies have been collecting all sorts of information for some time, and have now crept over into the patient's constitution, doing cholesterol levels perhaps and things like that. It may be impossible to put back the clock with respect to individuals' height, weight and so on, but if a line has to be drawn, I think it could probably be justified to draw it at the genotype. If we start looking at the DNA, there would be good reasons for drawing the line there rather than elsewhere.

Austin: With regard to homosexuality, if it were proved that there is a biological factor which influences homosexuality and if genetic screening were introduced (because it is shown that homosexuals are probably more likely to contract AIDS since there is a higher prevalence in their community), that information should also be given to the insurers. The people who would be making the decisions about whether to operate to remove that condition, or whether an abortion should be performed would be heterosexuals, because heterosexuals, by and large, are the people who are reproducing. Would that be ethically correct?

Genetic screening-1

PATRICK NAIRNE [1]

The Nuffield Council on Bioethics has fifteen members, of whom only seven are scientists or clinically qualified. My task, together with Mrs Caroline Miles, is to present the report of the Council, *Genetic Screening: Ethical Issues* (hereafter, *GSEI*) [2].

Genetic screening has been with us for some years. For 20 years in the United Kingdom, newborn babies have been screened for a rare inherited disorder, phenylketonuria, and for some years there have been pilot screening studies for monogenic diseases, in particular cystic fibrosis. The Human Genome Project, can be expected to lead to widespread genetic screening including the difficult field of polygenic diseases. There is therefore an urgent need to introduce effective and acceptable safeguards, standards and procedures relating to informed consent, counselling and confidentiality, and to the risk of discrimination in employment and insurance. There is a parallel need to stimulate wide public discussion and debate about the social and ethical consequences and questions that touch us all. That, put briefly, is the message, fully endorsed by the Nuffield Council, of *GSEI*.

---

1. Chairman of the Nuffield Council on Bioethics. Formerly Permanent Secretary Department of Health and Social Security.
2. Available from the Nuffield Council on Bioethics, 28, Bedford Square, London, WC1 3EG.

In considering the ethical implications of genetic testing and screening, it has to be kept in mind, first, that about three in every 100 children are born with a severe disorder presumed to be genetic or partially genetic in origin; and secondly, that genes often linked with environmental factors are being identified as a contributory factor of many common diseases such as coronary artery disease, some cancers, diabetes and Alzheimer's disease.

In broad terms, what emerges from *GSEI* is that genetic screening does not raise any entirely new ethical issues, but the problems it poses for individuals screened or tested, for their families, for health care professionals, and for society at large, can be more complex and difficult than those now encountered in most areas of clinical treatment. It is clear that the introduction of population-based screening for genetic diseases will require not only additional resources, but also ethical sensitivity, for example, in securing informed consent.

The Report's introduction explains (1.13): "Throughout our report we have kept in mind two fundamental points on the ethics of health-care decisions. First, there may be certain courses of action that should be ruled out whatever their seeming benefits. In the context of genetic screening we emphasize that compulsion should be ruled out... Second, the question must always be posed: does the potential good outweigh the possible harm?"

To take a simple example, if a family has a medical history of the rare disorder, Huntington's disease, would younger members of the family wish to be screened? They may see no potential benefit when there is no therapy. They already face potential insurance difficulties. They may also foresee harm to their careers if employers were to require a health check which yielded a positive result of a genetic test years in advance of the symptoms of the disease emerging. On the other hand, the younger members of the family might wish to accept the risk of a test in the hope that it would prove negative, so removing fears relating to employment or insurance and to their transmission of the disease to the next generation.

When genetic screening becomes available for polygenic diseases the difficulties of assessing the genetic susceptibility of individuals are likely to make it even more ethically important to respect the autonomy of the individual — an autonomy individuals must be empowered to express by way of informed consent, or informed refusal, when screening or testing is offered.

Although I hesitate to speak about justice in the presence of some distinguished lawyers, it is of great importance in relation to genetic screening. As I understand it, the formal principles of justice state that each person must be given his or her due, and that equals must be treated equally. That immediately poses the questions: are not a job and life insurance each person's due, irrespective of his or her circumstances? Does the concept of equals being treated equally make any sense if everyone's genetic make-up is different, with a different effect on health and life?

These are not easy questions and I wish to end my address with a few words about the Council's conclusions relating to insurance, employment and (especially) public education.

Chapter 6 is on employment. The Working Party found no evidence in the United Kingdom of uses of genetic screening by employers which should concern us at present. As genetic screening becomes more widely available, employers may, however, seek to require screening for some occupational diseases, or where there is any likelihood that an employee's illness or condition will present a danger to other employees. So a more stringent approach to occupational disease, assisted by a wider use of genetic test information, ostensibly in the interests of employees, could lead to discrimination against those with adverse test results.

In the view of the Nuffield Council, this is essentially a health and safety issue: *i.e.* people should be excluded from employment opportunities only where this is shown to be absolutely necessary on health and safety grounds.

Paragraph 6.28 summarizes the strict conditions which, in the Council's view, must be met before genetic screening of employees should even be contemplated. This, the Council suggests, is the right approach at present; we recommend that the Department of Employment keep the matter under review. The problems of insurance, on the other hand, are already with us, and urgent. Families with a history of serious disease can experience significant insurance problems now. What has been forecast about the wider use of genetic screening, particularly as it may be applied to those with genetic susceptibilities, has naturally aroused anxiety about insurance discrimination in the future, especially among those for whom house purchase and life insurance go together; and, for individuals who have an essential need for insurance, it is a matter of justice that there should be adequate safeguards.

Chapter 7 of *GSEI* clarifies important differences in assessing insurance risks between (a) dominant disorders (*e.g.* Huntington's chorea) and recessive disorders (*e.g.* cystic fibrosis); and (b) monogenic disorders (Huntington's chorea and cystic fibrosis) and the polygenic disorders where genetic susceptibility is just one factor predisposing to the disorder. It is the latter, the polygenic and multifactorial diseases, which will present the greatest problem. This is because of the difficulty of assessing in any individual what may be slender evidence of his or her susceptibility to develop later in life one of these polygenic diseases when account is taken of environmental and wider health factors. Of course, the insurance industry and their medical advisors understand all this.

The Council report made clear that insurance companies should receive the results of any relevant genetic test where there is a family medical history which would be disclosed at present, and also where an application is made for an insurance policy of more than moderate size.

The insurance industry, for its part, has given assurances that it does not intend to ask for genetic tests when an insurance application is received. However, as I think might be expected, the industry is most reluctant at present to accept that anyone who has undergone genetic screening should not disclose the result, even though there is no relevant family history, and the policy application is of a straightforward and moderate character.

This is a serious issue, potentially for all of us, and for the underwriters, and led to the Council recommendation that the best course at this stage will be to establish a temporary moratorium during which the United Kingdom Government and the insurance industry should discuss the future use of genetic information. (The Netherlands has experience of this.) I would like to think that this may be the start of a continuing dialogue between the government and the insurance industry in which they keep under joint review the development of genetic screening and its implications for insurance over the years ahead.

That is all I want to say by way of outlining the major features of the report with important social implications other than those which Mrs Miles will address. In conclusion, first, I would like to stress again the uncertainties we now face. Even with greater medical knowledge, there may be wide margins of error in assessing from a genetic test the risks affecting individuals and their families. This accentuates the ethical dilemmas which individuals and their families, with some professional help, may have to resolve, and the ethical problems or potential problems in employment and insurance which I have briefly summarized.

No report can offer a kind of ethical "cookbook" in which an index will point the way to ethical recipes for every question that may arise, but we hope that the Nuffield Council report will lead to the establishment, in this country, of a framework of safeguards, standards and procedures that will enable people both to answer the questions for themselves, and to reach the decisions which are important to them.

Secondly, there are measures which governments with the assent of parliaments — not only, I suggest the United Kingdom Government and the Parliament — must adopt, and responsibilities they must exercise in order to ensure that professional staff, employers and the insurance industry respond effectively to ethical requirements that must be met.

But that is not enough. The ethics of genetic screening is not just a challenge for others. It is a challenge for us all. Chapter 8 of the report brings out the important need for much better public understanding of human genetics — a crucial safeguard against stigmatization and the possible risk of abuse. The media obviously have an important and responsible role, so have schools and colleges. As I think everyone will agree, we who are concerned with the ethical and social consequences have to accept our responsibilities, recognizing that we are now only on the threshold of the range of ethical problems which further scientific developments may bring.

Genetic screening-2

CAROLINE MILES[1]

I begin with two general points. First, the Nuffield Council is not a government-sponsored body. It has been established by one of the major charitable foundations in the United Kingdom, with the object of promoting and encouraging informed debate on difficult ethical issues at the frontiers of medical science. Secondly, in the Working Party on genetic screening we were not concerned with screening as an aspect of research into the causes and treatment of genetic disorders, although we recognize that information collected when screening people in clinics may be useful for research. We also did not consider the ethical aspects of screening as a means of obtaining statistical information about the prevalence and distribution of disease-linked genes. In other words, we were not concerned with anonymous screening for genetic defects. This is an important point in relation to the whole question of confidentiality and consent.

The Working Party was therefore looking at the clinical aspects of screening for genetic disease; and I should add that we were focusing on serious diseases (from Huntington's disease, or Duchenne muscular dystrophy, to cystic fibrosis and

---

1. Member of the Nuffield Council. Formerly chaired the Oxford Health Authority.

the haemoglobin disorders such as sickle-cell disease and thalassaemia).

There is a variety of mechanisms by which serious genetic diseases are inherited. There are the dominant genes, where, in fact, an individual with the gene is very likely to develop the disease, and the recessive genes, where essentially both parents must have the gene for their offspring to develop the disease. On the other hand, an individual may be a carrier of the defective gene and never develop the disease. Going further, there are obviously difficulties about both the accuracy of testing and the predictability of somebody who has a potentially serious gene actually developing the disease, and how severely. All these risks and uncertainties surrounding so much of medical genetics still remain, as Sir Patrick has already emphasized.

With regard to consent, even within the context of ordinary medical treatment, there is still considerable discussion, in the United Kingdom and elsewhere, about what constitutes adequately informed consent. There are differences of view amongst both doctors and patients as to what information constitutes adequate information, and in particular how to understand the possible range of outcomes of a disease or a treatment for a disease, and the risks associated with specific treatments.

There are two additional problems with genetic screening. First, with screening, and in particular screening for recessive genes (where the individual does not know that he or she has a family history of anything), an individual who feels perfectly well, and indeed is well, is approached out of the blue by a health care professional and asked whether he or she wishes to be tested for the presence of a particular gene. If this gene is found to be present, it may mean that the individual will develop a fatal condition or, more likely, carries a gene which, if he or she decides to have a child with somebody who also carries the gene, will mean that their child will have a serious risk of developing a genetic disease — most of the genetic diseases still being incurable. In contrast with the information a sick patient needs to give consent to medical treatment, the information sought by a healthy individual considering whether or not to be screened is, then, presented in a setting which exposes a wide range of issues. This includes questions beyond those about the nature and severity of the disease, possible treatments and so on, such as:

1. Will everybody who has the faulty gene develop the disease?

2. How severely will they develop it?

3. How significant are environmental factors and the presence of other diseases?

We are then of course getting into the area of polygenic diseases and genetic predispositions to develop common diseases. (In GSEI (para. 4.8), there is a list of the kinds of information which, it seemed to us, is essential for informed consent, and so, to make an autonomous choice to be screened for a genetic disease.)

The second key difference between screening for genetic disease and the "ordinary" medical encounter relates to the consequences of a genetic test for families. Here, we are on parallel ground as testing for HIV. If someone is found to carry a defective gene, there will be a predictable chance of that individual's brothers and sisters, and indeed more remote relations perhaps, also carrying the gene. The Council felt that family members therefore have a legitimate and strong interest — I avoid the word "right" — in knowing the results of that person's test, because it may also affect them, their own family, and their reproductive decisions.

We have stressed in the report the importance attached by the Nuffield Council to ensuring that, before agreeing to be tested, people have thought through their relationships with other family members, and the problems with which they may have to cope and think about if they decide to have children. We argue that this is all part of informed consent.

I now turn to issues raised by counselling and confidentiality. The Council feels that adequate counselling is important but, on such evidence as we were able to obtain from pilot studies, this does not necessarily mean extensive face-to-face discussions. It means giving careful thought to the kind of literature (leaflets) given to people, deciding when it would be right to suggest that they might like to be screened, which will be when they have a real interest in, and motivation to understand the purpose of the screening. I would see counselling at the edge of, but an important part of broader education and the development of public understanding of what medical genetics is all about and where it is taking us.

As I have already said, given the importance of the familial dimension of genetic screening, it follows that the issues of consent and confidentiality are essential. How do we then take account of what are clearly the legitimate interests of close family members? We discussed, at some length, the question of making this information available to family members automatically in some way. We felt this would be deeply wrong because it would run counter to the basic principle of confidentiality. Provided that people have understood the purpose of screening, we felt that almost all of them (probably more than 99%) will understand the importance of sharing the information with their family members. There may be very rare instances (we found one or two examples, quoted in the report) in which the doctor may feel that it is his duty to override the wishes of the person who has been screened and tell immediate family members even if someone says that he or she absolutely does not want his brother, sister or whoever to know. We have suggested that this is a matter that needs to be discussed by the professional standard setting bodies of the medical profession — and the nursing profession — with a view to providing guidelines to doctors and nurses.

One other point on confidentiality to which the Working Party gave some thought is whether the existing statutory protection of medical information in the United Kingdom will be adequate. (All information stored on a computer is protected in the United Kingdom under the existing Data Protection Act (1984), which provides for the registration and supervision of data users. To obtain registration, a user must name all those to whom it is intended to disclose the data, which, then, may not be disclosed to others after registration.) We felt, first, that this is an area government should look at, to make sure that the existing law is adequate. Secondly, it is important to make clear to people, when they are considering whether to be screened, that they would have a right to request that the sample be destroyed as soon as the test which was the immediate purpose of taking the sample has been performed. I make this point because most people's medical records have blood spots on them, taken years before, which could be, and have been, used at any time to examine the composition of their DNA.

Finally, a brief comment on our suggestion as to the way in which genetic screening might be introduced and monitored in the United Kingdom as a clinical service. I suspect that some of the Europeans present may regard it as a very British way of doing things, but I think it does work. We have suggested that government should consider, through some enabling legislation, setting up a co-ordinating and monitoring body. This body should monitor screening programmes once they are in place to make sure that they are: (1) following proper standards and criteria in providing information to people; (2) not introducing an element of compulsion; (3) protecting the data; (4) following any guidelines and rules that have developed in relation to the release of data for insurance. The relevant body should also assess, and recommend to government, the value of establishing a screening programme before its inception.

In our view, a genetic screening programme should be introduced in the clinical setting only if it can be shown to be of net benefit to the people who will be screened and their immediate families. In particular a monitoring body should consider:

— the predictive power and level of accuracy of the test;
— the value to those being screened of the knowledge;
— the availability or otherwise of therapy for the condition (which does not necessarily mean that the lack of any therapy makes the screening not worthwhile);
— the potential social implications;
— the resource costs.

That is all I want to say about the Nuffield report. I make two brief points in conclusion. First, there are ethical issues in common between HIV screening and screening for genetic diseases, not least the question who should share the information obtained through screening. There are, however, some key differences, one of which is the way in which these diseases are transmitted. Our approach to educating and helping people to think about their own responsibilities in relation to HIV is extremely different from the proper approach to understanding the implications of having a genetic disease or a disease-indicating gene. This follows through into the area of consent, of education, of the confidentiality of the information, and so on[2].

Secondly, in the context both of HIV and of genetic disease, there is the danger of losing sight of the primary purpose of any such screening; this purpose is ultimately to benefit the individuals, the people who are suffering or who may suffer from the disease and their families, their immediate social network. In the areas of genetics and of HIV, if we ever get beyond that and ask whether some greater society good would be achieved by doing something, even if it is gravely damaging to individual people, this should be ruled out on the grounds spelled out in our report that some things should not be done because they are morally wrong.

---

2. Screening does not always come at people in this way. There are people with family histories of genetic disease; and there is also widespread testing of women during pregnancy and of newborn babies, both in this country and throughout much of the world now, for a number of conditions of genetic origin. The table on p. 27 of GSEI lists the screening that now goes on in the United Kingdom.

Invited response

LUDGER HONNEFELDER [1]

I want to acknowledge the excellent report of the Nuffield Council and Working Party. The report states, with good reason, that the legitimacy of genetic screening depends upon each patient's medical counselling, the indication of a serious disease, and informed consent. If a person's identity is largely determined by genetic design, and is protected by integrity and dignity, a line has to be drawn with regard to diagnosis and therapy which afford protection to this identity.

The following questions arise: How can diseases that fall within the category for which broad screening is allowed, be prevented from becoming conditions which cause people to feel that sufferers should be avoided, or are health-politically unwanted? To cite the report of the German Federal and State-Level Working Party on Genome Analysis, is there a chance that a genetic aberration could be qualified as a disease "without regard to its individual form in each affected person"? How shall we prevent the stigmatization of those who suffer from diseases which seem to be avoidable? (This is "eugenics from below", as stated in the final report of the TA project on genome analysis of the Technology Assessment Unit of the German Bundestag.)

---

1. Professor of Philosophy, Rheinische Friedrich-Wilhelms Universität Bonn.

These difficulties with genetic screening are seen in connection both with the monogenic diseases which begin later in life and cannot be cured by treatment, and with the diseases diagnosed prenatally, which cannot be prevented except by abortion — a solution that "prevents a disease by preventing the individual himself", as one German geneticist has put the matter.

How can judgements about life that is worth living and life that is not worth living, and the related selection of unborn life, be avoided? In German law at present, abortion is justified only if the birth of a severely genetically affected child is not acceptable to the mother; it cannot be justified by the claim that the genetic handicap is judged unacceptable to the unborn child; and in 1989 the German Bundestag followed the advice of the Enquete-Kommission in "Opportunities and Risks of Gene Technology", and passed a resolution disapproving the screening of non-curable diseases such as muscular dystrophy.

*
* *

Discussion [2]

Administrative and technical issues

Fluss: What happens now to a report such as this? What is the likely approach of the Department of Health and other

---

2. Once again comments and questions are collected into three broad, overlapping categories, namely: (1) the administration of, and technical issues arising from genetic screening programmes; (2) access to screening data by employers and insurance companies; (3) practical and ethical problems relating to those screened and their kin, including unborn children. These are followed by a (4) general discussion.

government departments which are addressed by particular recommendations?

Secondly, with regard to the co-ordinating body mentioned in Chapter 9, are there any alternatives to legislation, given the difficulties in getting legislation in these areas in the UK? Would it not be simple for government to establish a working party such as those set up to discuss issues of gene therapy?

Nairne: Before the report was published, advance copies were sent to the Department of Health and to all the other government departments concerned. We discussed the recommendations informally with the higher reaches of the Department of Health. That Department would not of course give us, as an independent body, any assurances as to how their ministers would act, but they certainly left us with the impression that the report's conclusions and recommendations would be taken very seriously.

There has already been parliamentary interest. At least one MP has taken up the report with ministers of various departments as well as the Department of Health — the Department of Employment and the Department of Trade and Industry, which has some interest in insurance. I would hope that both the House of Commons and the House of Lords will follow this up and take a close interest in it.

On Mr Fluss' second question, it is not certain that it will be necessary to set up a statutory body as a co-ordinating body; it may well make sense to start with an advisory body, see whether that is effective. If I were still the Permanent Secretary at the Department of Health, I would expect to have a full consultation process with the health authorities, the Royal Colleges and professional representatives on the suggestions we have made, and the proposals about setting up a co-ordinating body. In the light of that process, I would hope that within the course of a year, perhaps sooner, there would be a decision to set up a body which might be advisory at the start.

Miles: I agree; if, after a consultation process (which might involve discussion in both Houses of Parliament, as well as public discussions of the kind we are having today), the government of the day decided a statutory body was necessary, I do not think it would be elaborate legislation. It would probably be uncontentious legislation that would get on the statute book relatively quickly.

Nairne: The media have asked me whether the Nuffield Council gains by being a body independent of government, or whether effective action on the conclusions and recommendations would be more likely if we had been set up by government. (I would not say that we are unique, but in most other countries bodies doing similar work are established by government.) It is a nicely balanced question. Governments often set up inquiries, and do not like the conclusions or recommendations, or decide there are more important bits of government business to get on with — and do not always act on them. On the other hand, if they have set up the body themselves, they are likely to be pressed rather more closely as to what action they are taking. Against that, we have possibly gained in authority by being independent of government in the work we are doing.

De Wachter: When we talk about pregnancy-screening, do we mean screening of both parents at the same time?

Miles: It depends on all sorts of things — for example, on what is being screened for. In pilot studies, sometimes both partners have been offered screening simultaneously. Sometimes only the mothers-to-be are offered screening, and then if they are found to have the relevant gene, partners are then offered screening. This is still very much at a trial stage.

Holm: Mrs Miles says [in section (2) below] that it is possible to screen during pregnancy, but also earlier — citing evidence that schoolchildren accepted screening. Can she expand on that, and upon what sort of weight could be put on the acceptance of screening by schoolchildren?

[Mrs Miles referred the question to Dr Anionwu.]

Anionwu: I can give two examples, one in the United Kingdom that was negative, and one in Montreal on Tay-Sachs that was positive. The negative one was a project in Luton. The people who carried it out argued that, because it was possible to offer prenatal diagnosis for the haemoglobinopathies, would it not be a good idea to provide information and offer screening within a school in an area where there were ethnic minorities? In fact, the article gave the impression that that was successful.

The criterion for success was the number of carriers identified with haemoglobinopathies and glucose-6-phosphate dehydrogenase deficiency (which was also included). I must stress that it is very much my personal opinion that it was a negative study. I wondered whether it was successful because there was the comment that the only negative result in terms of the response was in a girl described as a teenager of West Indian origin who reacted in a stigmatized fashion, but that there were known social problems with this girl (these may not be the exact words).

The Tay-Sachs experience, on the other hand, is wedged within a whole history of community education and involvement with the relevant organizations, with a background of thought into the information programme.

Marteau: In *GSEI* it is clear that one of the primary objectives of genetic screening is to provide information to the people who come forward for screening. If that really is the objective, our screening programmes should be evaluated and the results reported in that kind of way.

Given the criteria set out for thinking about genetic screening programmes, and given the important distinction between offering screening and treatment, might there be some advantage in the advisory body considering not just genetic, but all screening programmes?

Miles: I think there is something to be said for having a body which evaluates all screening programmes; one of the advantages of having a National Health Service (NHS) is that it ought to be possible to do it. In the NHS, about ten years ago, screening for cervical cancer was introduced in an unsystematic way: different age groups of women, different periods between calling back for re-screening in different parts of the country, and so on. This caused great distress, much though not all of it unnecessary if the programme had been thought out.

Young: Why was *GSEI* not concerned with screening either for research or for statistical purposes? I suggest that what is left (the medical aspects of screening) is not a real subject. Given that many underlying genetic conditions are ripened into the actuality of disease only by an environment, the public health authorities will need to know the prevalence of those susceptibilities in order to manage and plan health provision in general. If the doctors and counsellors are to counsel people they surely need to know as much as possible both about the prevalence of the condition and the effects on it of certain environments.

Miles: We looked at applications of genetic screening in medical practice because those were our terms of reference, and I think it is the aspect of the matter that most urgently needs thinking about. One of our basic principles is that the leading purpose of screening in medical practice is to benefit the person being screened, not just to collect information. It is never clear what we would do with the information until a later stage, but the possibility that the information gathered in this way may be useful for other purposes is not excluded.

Practical and ethical problems relating to those screened and their kin, including the unborn

Nairne: A number of issues lie at the centre of this topic, one of which is the ethical question of the right of an individual to choose whether a child should be born when it is known that the child may be born with a genetic defect or disease. Against that, is the question of whether there are any limits to the choice of the individual. I think it is difficult to say categorically that there are no limits. If we say there are limits, what are they? Do they arise from the resource costs? These are problems for public discussion.

Miles: It would be mistaken to assume that the only point at which it is possible to screen is during pregnancy, for it is feasible to screen schoolchildren. (This is already a part of some screening programmes, certainly for sickle-cell disease in some countries.) It appears from one or two reports I have read that schoolchildren understand what screening is all about, and accept it.

This is obviously a different kind of a choice from the choice to have an abortion. I think it would be a pity to focus too much on whether screening should be allowed, depending on one's views on abortion.

Harris: As I understood it, Professor Honnefelder endorsed the quotation that it is wrong to prevent the disease by preventing the patient; that, we most effectively do by screening would-be parents and leaving them the decision as to whether to procreate. As technology advances, it may be possible to screen the gametes, not the embryo, before conception with the possibility of the same consequence, namely, preventing the disease by preventing the patient. Does Professor Honnefelder regard both of these practices as intrinsically wrong for related reasons?

Secondly, in cases where genetic information about one family member has important consequences for another, *GSEI* couches its advice in conditional terms: if a patient declines to impart the information to family members, this *may* (not must) be overridden. In couching the advice in this gentle conditional way, I wondered why the interests of the screened patient were prioritized over the interests of the other family members, and whether Mrs Miles really thinks that such prioritization is legitimate.

Miles: At that point in the report, we were speaking generally about whose claim to autonomy, whose interest should prevail over who else's interest. I cannot see any answer, "generally speaking", to that question, so I think it will depend, to some extent, on the nature of the disease being screened for, and on the statistical predictability of siblings and other blood relations being affected by the same gene. There is a serious difficulty here, which I admit we have slightly fudged.

Nairne: I agree with Mrs Miles. There may, for example, be a situation in which some of the family who would be affected are in Australia. The individual who has been screened for something that is late onset may say he is not in touch with them, he could not worry them, has not seen his sister for 30 years, and so on. There are enough individual factors that may arise in addition to what may be called the "clinical factor" for the word "may" to be the correct word in this context.

Super: To comment on Professor Honnefelder, if we indulge in carrier screening for any genetic disorder, we are an accessory before the fact when couples decide to take the information and terminate a pregnancy.

I was very interested in *GSEI*, but there seems to have been a neglect of one aspect in which I have been involved. There has been only passing reference to the involvement of other members of the family. In one of the leaflets about screening offered during pregnancy the question is put, "shall I tell other members of my family? It is up to the individual, but other family members of child-bearing age may like to know".

In the North-West health region from April 1993 carrier screening has been funded for the families of people with cystic fibrosis. When the cystic fibrosis gene was discovered in 1989 there was no controversy about the need to offer carrier screening to family members — it was taken for granted that family members would be interested in knowing.

Since 1989, we have told people that we would test any family members who would like to be tested. From April 1993, we have indulged for the first time in active cascade carrier screening, which means that we have worked through the families. By telling people about the existence of the screening and encouraging them to make contact with their relatives, the latter have been approaching us. Between 1989 and April 1993, 500 relatives of people with cystic fibrosis were tested. Since April 1993 another 800 have been tested, so there has been a great increase in the interest as a result of us being active.

It might be asked whether we should be so active? Nobody is coercing anybody to be tested. People are being made aware of the offer of testing. Our predictions of the uptake are that 20 family members per family will be interested in being tested. There is a very high possibility of detecting carrier couples: in fact the rate of detecting them is ten times higher than with unfocused screening. There is also more meaningful reassurance to the majority of couples who test negative. Reassurance to people who know something about the disease is more meaningful than unfocused screening.

There has been intensive use of the information. We have tested 1,500 relatives so far, and have detected 15 carrier couples. Of the nine pregnancies in those 15, eight had prenatal diagnosis, and in four of the instances in which cystic fibrosis was predicted, three of the couples terminated the pregnancy.

If the testing of families and relatives were to be adopted, during the next 2-3 years the important education process could be more in place (I do not think it is at the moment, in terms of people coming forward for screening). This process could then be reduced, as it is in Toronto and in Montreal in the case of Tay Sachs disease, where every Jewish person now knows of the existence of these tests, and nobody needs to campaign any more: those who want the test come forward to have it. That would be the ideal way, but we are not quite ready for it in the United Kingdom. We need to be a little more active in making contact with families.

Nairne: That is most interesting. Were those families all approached personally or were they responding to something that they read? Secondly, where did they go for the testing and, thirdly, what proportion of people, when contacted, refused to have the test?

Super: We have been keeping a register of cystic fibrosis in the North-West for about the last six years. We know about all the children and adults with cystic fibrosis in our region, and also about all the paediatricians and physicians who care for people with cystic fibrosis. When we were funded, I wrote to them in the first instance and invited them to discuss with their cystic fibrosis patients the fact that we had been funded to do this particular work. They were then invited to send through the names to us. We were sent 500 names, a good proportion of whom were known to us already because of our work on DNA analysis over the years up to the discovery of the gene.

The understanding in my letter to the paediatricians and physicians was that we would have their blessing on us knowing the names of those people, who would then be contacted by us. The 500 people were sent a circular letter, saying that it would take us a long time to get round to all of them, and that those who had relatives who might be planning a family might wish to make themselves known to us sooner rather than later. A field worker was appointed for this particular work. She either visits people, or reacts to a dedicated phone call, and gives them mouthwash bottles; the samples are then sent to us.

We are aware of 11 nuclear families who were not interested. We know of some relatives (often it seems to be an individual family member) who, when contacted, have sent us enormous family trees. There are others who, after being contacted, say they do not feel like having the test — of course, no pressure is put on them.

Walton of Detchant: With regard to screening in the broad sense, society and the United Kingdom Department of Health have recognized for many years the importance of screening neonates for the presence of diseases such as phenylketonuria (PKU) and congenital hypothyroidism, because these conditions, once detected, can be effectively treated. There has, however, been a reasonable, and I think natural, resistance to screening neonates for diseases which can be identified at that age but which cannot subsequently be effectively treated. One example is Duchenne muscular dystrophy. It is now possible to detect all such cases at birth, and pilot studies have shown that a screening programme is perfectly reasonable, but as yet, although treatment with gene therapy may be not too far away as a result of recent research, there is no effective treatment. Another problem is that thousands of newborn boys have to be screened with a simple blood test to pick up a single case. I used to believe that it was not cost-effective to carry out such a screening programme, but now, I believe it is. One difficulty is that, in such a family, a second, or even a third affected child may often be born before the disease is diagnosed in the first-born, which, I think, is a powerful justification for such a programme in terms of preventive medicine.

Most single gene diseases for which genetic screening is now possible are rare, but let us consider a recent discovery relating to the apolipoprotein gene, *Apo-E4*. (I think this was published after *GSEI* appeared). It is not yet certain, but people who are homozygous for the *Apo-E4* gene seem to have a high probability of developing Alzheimer's disease in their 50s and 60s. It is horrifying to contemplate employers and insurance companies getting hold of that information. What is the attitude of the speakers to this problem — to individuals who learn of this and say that they must be tested to see whether they are homozygous for this gene because they want to know whether or not they will lose their mind when they are 50 or 60?

Miles: These matters were discussed a little in the Working Party. It would not be totally untrue to say that we backed out of them to some extent. The information about early-onset Alzheimer's disease is very new and, as I understand it, the degree of predictability even of people who have this gene (or this particular bit of the genome's make-up) as well as the relative influences of the genetic and environmental factors are not very clear.

I take the point, though, with Duchenne muscular dystrophy. The members of the Working Party might have rather different views. I would be responsive to the point made by Lord Walton that parents who have had a baby boy who appears to be completely healthy but in fact carries that gene might want to know about it. The problem then is whether to screen every baby boy in the country or to ask parents whether there is a family history in the appropriate lines of the family and then offer screening to those who have. This is a practical problem, and I am not sure about the solution. Lord Walton could tell us how straightforward and how reliable the test is. I can certainly see the long-term advantage. I am thinking of one or two particular cases of people who have wanted to know because they could then find out in subsequent pregnancies whether or not the foetuses carry the same gene.

Nairne: It is always enormously helpful and informative to hear Lord Walton speak on such matters as muscular dystrophy.

From my departmental experience[3], I would say we have to wait and see. Pressures may build up from what might be called the "consumer", the Genetic Interest Group, who might feel it is important to have screening in this area. The professionals themselves, those who are deeply concerned with muscular dystrophy, may feel that knowledge is gaining ground in this area and that screening ought to be done. The Department would be aware of this, would want to discuss it with all the appropriate authorities, such as the Royal Colleges, and to consider the resource costs. It might then be introduced as a basis of policy guidance from the Department. It might be widespread, or begin in a much more selective kind of way. This is a rather rough-and-ready description of how these things may happen.

On the fascinating question of Alzheimer's disease, I am sure Lord Walton agrees that it must be open to an individual to ask for screening. Nobody is going to lay down the law and say someone must not go to his doctor and ask for the test. But I dare say that his clinical advisor, his GP, would probably not send him to a consultant to help him make up his mind, but almost certainly "counsel" him to think again in the light of the knowledge he is able to convey to him.

It is difficult to answer, but, in terms of the attitudes of the Working Party, the Nuffield Council or the Government, I do not think this is an area in which the Government will lay down the law straightaway.

Miles: Probably right now, in January 1994, they would not, but who knows where we will be by January 1996?

Dr Super said that the cystic fibrosis gene was discovered four years ago in 1989. First, if a couple decides to have a baby although they know it carries the gene, and the baby starts to develop the disease, the sooner the possibility is known about

---

3. Sir Patrick Nairne is a former Permanent Secretary (Director General) of the Department of Health.

and the more quickly the very effective therapies are introduced (although they are essentially palliative, in the sense that the disease cannot be cured) the better that child will do, surviving possibly into quite middle age with a good quality of life for much longer. Early knowledge is important.

Secondly, there seems to be now a real possibility that some form of somatic gene therapy for cystic fibrosis may become possible, in which case the screening situation would seem to me to be transformed for the better.

PKU, to which Lord Walton referred, is a good example of a very rare genetic condition which, if recognized at once and treated, can be effectively dealt with. It therefore seemed clinically advisable to the medical profession at the time that this should become a test universally given to all newborn babies. Although the number of cases detected is tiny, those cases can be effectively treated, so who knows where we will be with Alzheimer's in two or three years' time?

Screening data, employment and insurance

Frontali: There are a couple of points in the report that were not clear to me. First, screening for employment. Even within the limits imposed, I wonder whether the same recommendation for informed consent and autonomy of choice also holds for screening for employment? Informed consent to do a genetic test must be asked of the person seeking the job. If he refuses, is he losing the opportunity to get the job and, if so, where is the autonomy of his decision? There should be a little more thought on how screening for employment should be done in order to protect the individual.

Secondly, concerning insurance companies and the possibility of an individual being asked to disclose the results of any relevant genetic test when there is a family history of a serious genetic disease : does this mean that if in the past an individual has previously asked for a genetic test, say, for Huntington's disease, he is obliged to disclose the result, or that the insurance company may ask him to do the test ? In the first case, if an individual is asked to disclose a result already obtained, there will obviously be differences between people who ask for insurance having a similar family history, one of whom has previously had a genetic test and the other has not. What happens? Do they have different insurance policies? In the second case, if the insurance company is entitled to ask for the test to be done, again I think this affects the autonomy of the decision of the individual.

Nairne: More experience is needed on employment. That is really the thrust of what we say in the report. The only example quoted in the report of some form of genetic test is in the Royal Air Force where it is considered wise in relation to flying. As far as employees are more widely concerned, Dr Frontali raises a good point. All we have done so far is to specify conditions — very stringent conditions — that we believe should be met before an employer could even contemplate introducing genetic screening in relation to health and safety in the workplace. It might be interesting to hear the Danish experience on this, since, if I am right, Denmark has a draft Bill in relation to employment.

Our message is fairly simple on insurance: we have of course taken evidence from the Association of British Insurers, who have given an assurance that they will not ask for any genetic test to be done in response to an applicant applying for life insurance. At the moment, we take the view that, until these discussions that we are commending between government and insurers have taken place, it would be wrong for the insurance companies to make use of information from a test that has been done, though we have indicated the exceptions to that.

I am ready to be corrected, but my speculation is that those who have had tests are likely to be the same applicants as those who have a family medical history, which they would be disclosing anyway in accordance with normal practice for applicants applying for insurance in this country.

Miles: One point on screening by employers: as far as the United Kingdom is concerned, we are talking about the future. It is not happening now except in limited circumstances where it is for the protection, both of the employees concerned, and of other people. Airline pilots is one example.

More generally, in Paragraphs 6.18 and 6.19 of *GSEI*, we cite an example in the United States of America. In the early 1980s, a survey of a substantial number of large American companies showed that, whereas very few of them were testing for genetic diseases at that time, a considerable proportion said that they would be doing it within the next few years. However, when the survey was repeated six or seven years later, most of the companies had lost interest and were not contemplating genetic testing. I can only assume the reason is that they had decided it would not be cost-effective. Given the present state of knowledge of the nature and prevalence of genetic disease, I wonder how widespread genetic testing would become, simply on cost grounds.

Andersen: One recommendation of *GSEI* is to have a moratorium related only to screening or tests within the insurance field. Why distinguish between screening and tests with insurance and other applications? Has the possibility of a general moratorium been considered? The Danish Council of Ethics considered that it might be necessary to have a moratorium for some time on the whole field of genetic screening.

Nairne: Are you saying that there should be a moratorium on using any information, either for the individuals themselves or for research in that area? In the Nuffield Council's view, pilot screening programmes should make information available in the way described by Dr Super in respect of cystic fibrosis.

We saw no case for a moratorium in the field of employment; the evidence showed no reason for unease about genetic screening or genetic testing in respect of employment at present — but again we say that it should be kept under review.

Insurance, on the other hand, is a cause of anxiety now to those who have a family medical history arising from genetic causes. It has also been taken up by the media in the United Kingdom, in dramatized headlines and with comments about what may be emerging from the Human Genome Project and genetic research in this area. People are deeply worried — particularly those who seek to accompany their bid for house mortgages with life insurance — hence the moratorium and the discussions between government and industry.

Andersen: Within the clinical field, I think it is necessary to distinguish between two types of screening. First, screening in the strict sense: an offer of a test for a whole population or a defined part of a population. The common practice of prenatal diagnosis is screening in this strict sense. Secondly, screening for cystic fibrosis, another use of genetic diagnosis. There has been much discussion in Denmark about a pilot project of cystic fibrosis screening precisely because the then existing Danish Council of Ethics thought that this kind of screening was a crucial step further than the normal prenatal diagnosis. By a moratorium we mean that, at the moment, we do not want this kind of extension of the use of genetic diagnosis, for instance, in the sense of making it available for larger groups of individuals.

Young: To return to the matter of employers, were I going to work in the petrochemical or pharmaceutical industry, I would wish to be genetically tested before being employed in such a place, to be sure that I was not going to damage my own health or that of the fetus I might find myself carrying. I feel there is something back to front in looking at screening for employment as offensive to the individual's autonomy.

The role of the media

JOHN DURANT[1], ANDERS HANSEN[2]

The relationship between science (including medical science) and the mass media has been the subject of much comment and criticism over the years. Interestingly, two seemingly contradictory criticisms of mass media coverage of science are commonplaces. On the one hand, the mass media are often accused of distorting science through a coverage that is "inaccurate", "unbalanced", "sensationalist" or "scare-mongering"; and on the other hand, the mass media are often said to purvey a distinctly "uncritical" brand of science journalism that arises from an excessively close relationship between journalists and scientists. On the latter view, many science journalists tend to dispense with the role of public watchdog in favour of the role of public advocate on behalf of the scientific community. Either way, therefore, it would seem that, when it comes to science, the mass media simply cannot win. According to some critics, they are letting down the public by failing to fulfil their role as public watchdog.

The seemingly untroubled co-existence of these two apparently contradictory strands of criticism points to the need for

1. Professor of Public Understanding of Science at Imperial College, London, and Deputy Director of the Science Museum.
2. Centre for Mass Communications, Leicester University.

some careful thought about the relationship between science and the mass media. In this paper, we start by listing one or two fairly obvious but nonetheless easily forgotten features of the mass media and science; and then we go on to review briefly two particular examples of recent British mass media coverage of medical science; newspaper coverage of new developments in medical genetics; and newspaper coverage of HIV and AIDS. We suggest: first, that the issues raised by mass media coverage of medical science are complex rather than simple; second, that the problems raised by mass media coverage of science are not confined exclusively to the mass media themselves but rather embrace the scientific community as well; and third, that, in journalism as in science, very often the best remedy for bad professional practice is not censorship but rather the criticism that arises from good professional practice.

The mass media and Science

The "mass media" is a misnomer

The term the "mass media" is misleading, for it implies a homogeneous entity characterized by similar practices and objectives. It is doubtful whether this was ever the case; but whatever the situation may have been in the past, there can be no doubt that today, the umbrella term the "mass media" stands for an increasingly differentiated and complex system of agencies, institutions, processes and products.

A number of different distinctions are in order: distinctions between different kinds of media (print media, broadcast media, etc.); distinctions within particular kinds of media (tabloid newspapers, broadsheet newspapers, etc.); distinctions within specific media between different kinds of science coverage (news articles, feature articles, editorial comment, etc.); and so on. Particular media products may differ from one another in so many ways (medium, format, style, target audience, editorial stance, etc.) that it may be almost impossible to make direct comparisons between them.

Of special importance for present purposes is the distinction between science coverage in the mass media that is produced by specialist science journalists and broadcasters, and science coverage that is produced by general journalists and broadcasters. Specialist journalists are dependent upon the goodwill and continuing cooperation of the specific communities whose work they cover. This is especially true of specialist science journalists, who tend to have a particularly close relationship with professional scientists. Understandably, science journalists are anxious not to alienate their sources; and at the same time, they are usually keen not to incur the condemnation of their peers (Hansen, 1992). None of these constraints apply with anything like the same force to general journalists who happen to deal with science from time to time; and, for this reason, a more independent or even seemingly cavalier approach to scientific expertise is more likely from this quarter.

While it is important for an understanding of how science is covered in the mass media to appreciate the increasing differentiation which is taking place, it is also useful to acknowledge a parallel trend working in the opposite direction — namely, the increasing tendency of different media to "feed upon each other". The broadcast media frequently use press journalists as authoritative sources on science. Similarly, the popular press may take the broadcasting of a TV series as the occasion for launching their own discussion of a particular subject. For example, this has been the case in recent years in the fields of biotechnology and genetic engineering, with popular press coverage engaging with public hopes and fears aroused by television programmes such as *Chimera* and *The Cloning of Joanna May*.

"Science" is a misnomer

The term "science" is misleading in precisely the same way as the term the "mass media". Once again, the term "science" implies homogeneity and uniformity when, in reality, what we have to deal with is heterogeneous and varied. Two distinct kinds of variety are at work here. First, "science" is a label that stands for a wide variety of subjects — from astronomy to zoology. Second, "science" in the mass media may be taken narrowly to refer to the specialist coverage of science and scientific research, or it may be taken more broadly to refer to all coverage that refers to scientific matters. On the narrower view, we would find ourselves dealing principally with the specialist output of science journalists and broadcasters; but on the broader view, we would find ourselves dealing with a much larger and more varied output, embracing coverage labelled "Business", "environment", "health", and much else besides.

In studies of media coverage at the University of Leicester, one of us has found that something approaching one half of all portrayals of science or scientists in the mass media appear in articles or programmes which are not specifically about science at all. Science and scientists are drawn into a wide range of coverage, from crime and social problems to politics and consumer affairs. Precisely because it is not targeted at an audience that is already predisposed to be interested in science, it is likely that the scientific ideas and images incorporated into general media reporting of this kind are of great importance in the public domain.

Accuracy and distortion

There has been an enduring concern with the issues of "accuracy" and "distortion" in mass media coverage of science. For example, a series of American studies have surveyed scientists' assessments of the accuracy of stories in which they were quoted. Results from this type of research have varied. Some investigations have reported that scientists were generally satisfied with the accuracy of media coverage (*e.g.* Borman, 1978; Tichenor, Olien, Harrison and Donohue, 1970), while others have reported a high incidence of inaccuracies and errors (*e.g.*

Tankard and Tyan, 1974). It is possible that these very different results may reflect differences in research methodology (*e.g.* the types of questions asked) rather than differences in the accuracy of news coverage itself (Moore and Singletary, 1985).

A more basic problem with this type of research, however, is the concept of accuracy itself. What these studies tend to ignore, and consequently fail to throw much light on, is that there are fundamental differences between professional scientific communication and communication through the mass media. Scholarly publications must conform to a set of conventions and requirements that are quite different from those that apply to a newspaper or a popular magazine. If researchers set out to measure the performance of the mass media by the standards of scholarly publications (*e.g.* Singer, 1990), or even by the judgements of scientists themselves, then it is perhaps hardly surprising if they end up concluding that mass media coverage suffers from inaccuracies, omissions and other faults.

In a survey of more than 500 scientific or expert sources quoted in media science coverage, one of us has found that "accuracy" was rarely perceived as a great problem. Scientist sources for stories in the mass media tend on the whole not to be critical of the specific items of coverage in which they appear (*see also* Tichenor *et al.*, 1970). Of the 175 (*i.e.* about one third) of the sample who were sufficiently critical of the coverage to offer reasons for their dissatisfaction, only around one quarter complained that the coverage was factually inaccurate. In general, it is fair to say that the evidence from studies of this kind points strongly against the widespread existence of sloppy and distorted reporting.

There is one last and extremely important point to be made about accuracy. Very often, those who accuse the mass media of inaccurate science reporting conveniently ignore the fact that the media are reflecting uncertainties or even open disagreements within the scientific community itself. In such cases, one person's "inaccuracy" or "distortion" may be another's "accuracy" or "balance". Frequently, the mass media pick up on issues only after scientists themselves have "broken ranks" by raising difficulties, doubts or uncertainties. For example, the mass media gave relatively little coverage to the safety and morality of recombinant DNA technology until scientists themselves started drawing attention to these issues.

The linear model

According to the linear model of the relationship between science and the mass media, the scientific community produces knowledge (facts, findings, etc.) and the mass media then purvey this knowledge to the public in suitably shortened and simplified forms. Several things are wrong with this model. First, as we have already indicated, science is not always a source of uniformly unproblematic knowledge. In precisely those areas of science in which the mass media are most likely to be interested — *e.g.* new and path-breaking research, or socially relevant research —, there is likely to be doubt, uncertainty or even outright conflict within the scientific community (*see,* for example, Collins and Pinch, 1993). This obliges the mass media to make interpretive judgments about the reliability or validity of particular expert sources. Given the heterogeneity of the mass media, different media may be expected to make different interpretive judgments; and in extreme cases, there may even be open conflict within the mass media.

A second problem with the linear model is that it assumes that there is a clear distinction between science and the communication of science in the mass media. Increasingly, however, the mass media are caught up in the processes of science itself. Thus, it is not uncommon for scientists and scientific institutions to seek to exploit the mass media for their own ends (Nelkin, 1987; Hilgartner, 1989). One sign that this is happening is the increasing use of the mass media as a first outlet for new scientific results or claims. When this happens, the distinction between professional and popular scientific communication collapses; and a larger circle of critics and commentators is drawn into scientific debate. A good example here is the much-publicized debate about "cold fusion" in 1989; but other less high profile examples from the world of medical science also exist.

A third major problem with the linear model is that it presumes a passive and largely subservient role for the mass media. Although scientists and other professionals may wish to use the mass media for educational or even propagandist purposes, the mass media are not inherently educational or propagandist institutions. The owner and editor of a national newspaper, for example, are unlikely to view themselves first and foremost as educationalists; and even when they happen to be politically "aligned", they are unlikely to be willing slavishly to serve the perceived self-interest of a particular political party or group. Commercial, journalistic and other imperatives give the mass media a character that is quite properly distinct from the character of an educational institution or a public relations department; and this means that the mass media cannot realistically be contained within a simple, linear model of information transmission between the scientific community and the general public.

The impact of the mass media on the public

Finally, it is important to enter some caveats about the key question of the influence of the mass media upon the general public. Almost everyone who writes about our subject assumes that mass media coverage of science has important social effects. While we do not wish to deny this, it is important to observe that characterizing these effects is far from easy. For the past half century, mass communications researchers have sought to establish the relationship (if any) between media portrayal of violence and the incidence of violent behaviour in society. Though the questions are easy to ask, unambiguous answers have proved extremely elusive. There is no reason to suppose that establishing links between media coverage and public perceptions of science will be any less difficult.

In general, it seems fair to say that mass communications research has not demonstrated the huge and direct effects of the mass media upon the general public that are the stuff of social engineers' dreams. Research has rather tended to point to more specific and more localized influences which are mostly of an agenda-setting kind. Too often, discussion of mass media coverage of science operates with ill-defined notions of "the public"; indeed, the term "public understanding of science" suffers from the drawback that — naively interpreted — it appears to imply that there is one large homogeneous audience for science. In fact, it is far more instructive to consider the role of media coverage in relation to more clearly defined groups.

Perhaps the single most suggestive contribution to our understanding of the impact of mass media coverage of science on the public, at least for present purposes, is the work of Alan Mazur in the late 1970s (Mazur, 1981). Mazur studies the relationship between media coverage of scientific and technological issues and public perceptions of those issues. He found that the balance of negative and positive reporting seemed to have little measurable impact on people's perception of particular technologies. A deciding factor, however, was the extent to which a technology was portrayed as controversial. Mazur concluded that the presence of controversy generally made people more wary and suspicious of a particular science or technology. This is particularly relevant to the subject of screening for genetic disease or for AIDS, since these are topics which are often portrayed as subjects of scientific, moral and social controversy.

Media reporting on genetic disease

We have recently completed a study of British national newspaper coverage of genetic diagnosis and genetic screening, as part of a large study of the Human Genome Project and the British public for the European Commission (Durant *et al.*, 1993). The study made use of the electronic full-text database FT-Profile, which provides access to the following newspapers: *The Financial Times, The Guardian, The Times* and *The Sunday Times, The Daily Telegraph* and *The Sunday Telegraph, The Independent* and *The Independent on Sunday,* and *Today.* In addition, a manual search of the tabloid press was conducted. The study covered August and October 1991, and January-August (inclusive) 1992.

References to genes, genetics, biotechnology and/or DNA appear quite frequently in both the broadsheet and the tabloid press in Britain. Indeed, there is some evidence that coverage is increasing, particularly in the area of the mapping of the human genome, screening for genetic disorders and gene therapy. From the very outset in 1986, press coverage of the Human Genome Project has been dominated by a single set of questions and issues: the scientific significance of the project, the medical significance of the project, the commercial significance of the project (*e.g.* the patenting of DNA sequences), the costs of the project, the development of associated technologies (*e.g.* information technology), and last but not least, the considerable cluster of moral, legal, social and political issues that are raised by the project.

Several studies have noted the positive and relatively uncritical nature of news reporting on new genetic technologies (Nelkin, 1985; Nelkin, 1987; Goodell, 1986). What we found, however, was a pattern of reporting characterized by a mixture of two entirely different discourses: first, an enthusiastic, progressivist discourse centering on accounts of the great promise of genetic research for diagnosis and treatment (we shall refer to this as the "rhetoric of great promise"); and second, altogether less sanguine discussion of the many ethical, legal and social concerns that are raised by this area of research (we shall refer to this as the "rhetoric of concern"). During the period covered by our research, just over a third (34%) of all press articles mentioning research on the human genome made reference to ethical or moral issues.

Both the broadsheet and the tabloid press operated with the twin rhetorics of great promise and concern. Thus, on one occasion, the science correspondent of *The Financial Times* wrote that the Human Genome Project was "the largest international project in the history of biological research...The resulting 'Book of Man' may provide the basis for preventing or treating most human diseases in the next century" (*Financial Times*, 10 May 1989); but on another occasion, the same newspaper returned to the same subject under a headline with a very different tone: "The men who would play God: unravelling the secrets of the human gene could transform human life." But, as Clive Cookson reports, "the possibilities for abuse of this power are terrifying" (*Financial Times*, 1 February 1992). We note here, in passing, that of course science correspondents do not usually write the headlines under which their articles appear. This is yet another of the complexities that surround the coverage of science in the mass media.

Similarly, the tabloid press is capable of switching rapidly between the twin rhetorics of great promise and concern. Thus, we find articles with titles such as "The Positive Power of Gene Therapy — Genetic Manipulation as a Force for Good" (*Daily Mail*, 23 June 1992); but alongside such optimistic assessments are to be found altogether more sombre warnings, such as: "Your baby is going to be homosexual so we'll abort him: 'scientists' nightmare vision of DNA revolution" (*Daily Mail*, 12 May 1992), and a day later, "What Price will we Pay for these Medical Miracles?" (*Daily Mail*, 13 May 1992). "Nightmare vision", "Playing God", "Tampering with nature" and "Opening Pandora's Box" are metaphors that are commonly employed in the mass media as part of the rhetoric of concern. Images of "run-away" science, or of scientists as weird and sinister madmen, are actually few and far between in the British press. Two articles from our sample which came close to these stereotypes were actually concerned with the television play, *The Cloning of Joanna May*, by authoress Fay Weldon. Though these excited some critical comment from the scientific community, it is worth noting that in many ways they were the exceptions to the more general rule that tabloid newspaper coverage of genetic screening and gene therapy is dominated by the rhetoric of great promise. Where the coverage is concerned with forensic investigations of rape, murder or paternity, genetic finger-printing is generally portrayed as a unique, ingenious and infallible technique; and where it is concerned with medical issues, genetics is generally portrayed as a source of spectacular, life-enhancing or even life-saving diagnoses and treatments.

Having said this, we observe that, probably, the single most important area of moral and social concern in press coverage of genetics, in the period of this study, and more recently, has been the issue of the potential difficulties arising from the use of genetic information by insurance companies, potential employers and others. Here, where genetic discoveries raise the possibility of new and increasingly wide-ranging screening programmes for ever more genetic risk factors, the mass media are sustaining a debate which has wider resonances, not least with recent public debate about HIV and AIDS.

Media reporting of AIDS

AIDS has been one of the biggest medical stories in the British mass media over the past decade. As medical scientists unravelled the relationship between HIV and AIDS in the early 1980s, a remarkable consensus of scientific and medical opinion began to emerge. In brief: AIDS was a fatal infectious disease, caused by a "retrovirus" named HIV; HIV was transmissible by exchange of blood or other body fluids (including semen); identifiable "at-risk" groups included homosexual men who practised unprotected penetrative anal intercourse, people who injected drugs with previously used and unsterilized needles, and patients who may have been given transfusions of infected blood; and last but not least, although the bulk of early infections in the industrialized world were within "at-risk" groups, there was every likelihood that, in due course, the disease would spread to the general population, as it had already done in many parts of Africa. In short, AIDS was a major threat to public health; and in the absence of any immediate prospect of effective treatment, the most important task was to prevent the further spread of HIV infection through public health education — particularly about the importance of "safe sex".

Throughout the past decade, the mass media have generally cooperated with government, the medical community and the AIDS interest and support groups in spreading the word about HIV and AIDS. Faced with a new and potentially very serious public health issue, many of the mass media have seemed willing to adopt a "public interest" position not very far removed from that of, say, the Health Education Authority. Of course, mass media coverage of HIV and AIDS has not been confined to public health issues alone. Stories about scientific "breakthroughs" and setbacks, about the priority dispute between Robert Gallo and Luc Montagnier over who had priority in the isolation of the HIV virus, about prominent personalities who were HIV positive or who had AIDS, etc., have been given great prominence, particularly in the tabloid press; but for the most part, the British mass media have generally been content to follow the medical community in the way in which they have presented AIDS as a public health issue.

It is important, however, not to exagerate the extent and the uniformity of the consensus between the medical community and the mass media over AIDS. For example, in the 1980s, a number of tabloid newspapers suggested that AIDS was not a serious problem for the heterosexual community. These departures from the scientific and medical consensus were reinforced by the fact that some early predictions of the spread of HIV infection in Britain were proved to be too high. Of course, predictions of the spread of HIV are difficult and subject to multiple uncertainties, not least because of the impact of public health and public education campaigns themselves. Nonetheless, there is no doubt that among certain tabloid newspapers such as *The Sun*, lack of fit between forecasts and outcomes for the spread of HIV reinforced populist tendencies towards the scapegoating of particular minorities such as homosexuals and drug abusers.

In recent years, doubts about the scientific and medical consensus have spread beyond the tabloid press, and indeed into the broadcast media. A series of Channel 4 "Dispatches" programmes has openly questioned many elements within the conventional wisdom on HIV and AIDS; and a number of broadsheet newspapers have gone out of their way to promote what one national newspaper termed a "startling challenge to Aids orthodoxy" (*Sunday Times,* 26 April 1992). Sceptical articles and editorials in a number of newspapers over the past 18 months have cast doubt on the size of the threat posed by AIDS to the heterosexual community, the scale of the AIDS epidemic in Africa, and even the very existence of a causal link between HIV and AIDS. As one sceptical commentator put it in an article entitled "The unspoken truth on Aids", "virtually nothing told to us by the well-organized and lavishly financed Aids lobby has turned out to be true" (*Sunday Times,* 21 November 1993).

This sort of coverage has provoked a predictably strong reaction from the medical community, from AIDS interest and lobby groups, and from other sections of the mass media. There have been heated exchanges in the correspondence columns of *The Sunday Times*; and other newspapers (including *The Independent* and *The Daily Telegraph*) have voiced strong criticisms of the editorial line beting adopted by their sceptical journalistic colleagues. Where once the broadsheet newspapers spoke with an almost entirely united voice, we now have specialist science journalists openly at odds with one another, while one correspondent has written of *The Sunday Times* coverage of

AIDS over a period of 18 months that it is the product of "a kind of *folie à deux* between the editor and his science correspondent, a shared hysteria in the face of unfolding events" (James Fenton, *The Independent*, 6 December 1993). In the meantime, the Parliamentary Office of Science and Technology has responded to the debate by producing a briefing note for MPs on heterosexual AIDS, the opening paragraph of which reads as follows: Views in the media on the spread of HIV/AIDS among heterosexuals range from claims of a "plot" to overstate the risks, to warnings of a "ticking time bomb" with major implications for future public health. This is despite recent detailed information on HIV prevalence and sexual behaviour which allows more accurate projections to be made. (Parliamentary Office of Science and Technology, Briefing Note 46, October 1993.)

Is the emergence of scepticism about the "AIDS establishment" in certain sections of the British press simply the idiosyncratic result of a *"folie à deux"*? Or is it a symptom of deeper tensions in the relationship between medical science and the mass media? In order to answer this question, it is necessary to make a number of general points about recent media coverage of AIDS. First, it is worth recalling that AIDS is a disease of the mass media. The mass media have brought the problem of AIDS to the attention of the public; the mass media have facilitated the campaign by lobbyists in the gay community to obtain greater funding for AIDS research; the mass media have highlighted the urgency of the problem of AIDS by featuring prominent personalities who have been diagnosed as HIV positive; the mass media have sustained many of the larger fund-raising efforts that have helped to support AIDS research; and so on. Without the mass media, what the recent media critics refer to as the "AIDS industry" would scarcely exist.

Second, the emergence of dissenting voices in the mass media concerning AIDS cannot be attributed exclusively to the personal views of one newspaper editor and his science correspondent. Dissent has not been confined to *The Sunday Times*, or even to what is generally known as the "Murdoch Press". Over the past few years, other national daily newspapers have also published articles sceptical of one or another aspect of the orthodox medical view of AIDS. In addition, *The Sunday Times* has not spoken out uniformly against the medical consensus on AIDS. Over the past few months, articles that are implicitly or explicitly supportive of the orthodox view of AIDS have appeared in this newspaper as well as articles that are tacitly or explicitly critical of it. What we have to deal with, therefore, is not so much a personal *animus* against the orthodox view of AIDS (though of course such an *animus* may, in fact, exist) as a more general mass media climate of scepticism and uncertainty about the standard view of AIDS. As one newspaper put it, "*Today* does not claim that either side is right. What we do believe is that every avenue must be explored in finding a cure" (*Today*, 27 April 1992).

Third, it is vital to recognize that dissent from the standard view of AIDS did not originate in the mass media. In the late 1980s, the American virologist Peter Duesberg and others developed an increasingly sceptical view of the orthodox medical view of AIDS. Duesberg aired his views in conferences and occasional publications (Duesberg, 1987); and they were given further prominence by freelance journalist and author Jad Adams, in his book *AIDS: The HIV Myth* in 1989. By now, there was a fairly vociferous — if also fairly small — group of scientific sceptics who were prepared to challenge orthodoxy; and in the spring of 1992, a conference was organized in Amsterdam in order to give them a platform for their views. It is this conference which appears to have attracted the attention of sections of the British press to the existence of articulate opposition to the orthodox view of AIDS within the scientific community.

It seems, therefore, that we are dealing here with a decision by one section of the mass media to air a minority point of view within the medical community. As it happens, the broadsheet newspaper that has adopted the most consistently sceptical line on AIDS over the past two years — *The Sunday Times* — has a long and occasionally distinguished record of campaigning investigative journalism which includes a major contribution in the 1970s to the exposure of the thalidomide tragedy. Challenging the prevailing medical or scientific wisdom on the basis of careful and original investigation is an honourable journalistic strategy. In the present case, however, there appears to be little evidence of either care or originality in the sceptics' arguments; and, of course, the value of independent critical journalism must be weighed against the value of informing the public about potentially lethal health risks. Nevertheless, we would do well to reflect upon the fact that the argument about heterosexual AIDS was being prosecuted within the scientific community long before it was taken up in the mass media.

Conclusion

We started this paper with two seemingly contradictory criticisms of mass media coverage of science: first, the criticism that such coverage is inaccurate and distorted; and second, the criticism that such coverage is insufficiently independent of the views of scientists themselves. The two examples we have used illustrate some of the ways in which both of these criticisms may be valid. In the case of press coverage of genetic disease, we find that two completely different and largely unresolved rhetorics are employed — a rhetoric of great promise, and a rhetoric of moral concern. Both of these rhetorics are rather extreme, and it is very rare to find any attempt to reconcile them within a coherent account of the technical and the moral dimensions of medical genetics.

In the case of AIDS, we find some signs of the collapse of a medical and media consensus that, until recently, has dominated public discussion of the subject. The reasons for this collapse appear to lie in the growth of a minority point of view within the scientific community, coupled with what might be termed an ideological preference on the part of certain media to champion the cause of this particular minority in the face of the overwhelming majority view. Blanket scepticism about the entire edifice of scientific knowledge concerning HIV and AIDS is no more rational than blanket acceptance of it as absolute and timeless truth. Similarly, healthy journalistic independence does not involve simply signing up for one (minority) scientific point of view as opposed to another, but rather the critical weighing of different points of view. In the case of *The Sunday Times* and AIDS, it would seem that what started out as a desire to air a view that was not being voiced in public has become something of a crusade intended to confer legitimacy on that view.

Invited response

JOHN MADDOX[1]

I would like to put Professor Durant's description of the row between *Nature* and *The Sunday Times (ST)* in a slightly different form. First, our objection to the *ST* is not that it reported the heterodox view held by Peter Duesberg. It is, as Professor Durant said, that, as the months have gone by, their legitimate reporting of a dissenting view within the scientific community has been turned into a campaign which has been sanctimoniously likened to that newspaper's own successful and heroic campaign on behalf of the thalidomide people 20 years ago.

It seems to me wrong that a newspaper with many millions of readers should give exclusively one side of this complicated story, and dangerous that it should suppress the knowledge, that many of us believe to be useful, that HIV causes AIDS. We are not for censorship, which we believe is an even worse evil than that perpetrated by the *ST* in its line on AIDS; so we decided that *Nature* would monitor what the *ST* published about AIDS, week by week, and give its readers an account both of what the *ST* said and of the letters it was not publishing from correspondents who often found it extremely difficult to get their letters into the *ST*. The first response of the *ST* was an arti-

---

1. Editor of *Nature*; formerly Director of the Nuffield Foundation.

cle, headed "We Will Not Be Silenced", accusing *Nature* of trying to censor it.

Two matters in Professor Durant's paper disturb me. First, it began, perhaps overcynically, by saying that Tom Wilkie, of *The Independent*, had said to an audience like this that of course it must be remembered that the science journalist is there to sell newspapers. I do not believe this is true. None of the people who work as respectable science journalists on any European newspaper that I know of is there because he feels that it will add to the profits of the company that owns his newspaper.

Second, Professor Durant said in his paper that there was growing dissent about the orthodox view of HIV as a cause of AIDS. I do not believe this is true. There has been a rumble of dissent from Peter Duesberg over the past five years. At the outset, he made many friends in the AIDS community, and very few friends — or, rather, lost them — in the scientific community. As time goes on, Duesberg is increasingly isolated. People do believe that there is experimental and epidemiological evidence that HIV has something to do with AIDS. It is perverse, in my opinion, to suppose that this is a question yet to be decided.

One other point about genetics and screening that is relevant to some extent to AIDS is that geneticists themselves are sometimes guilty of gross oversimplification. For example, we all hear about "the cystic fibrosis gene". What is it? In fact, the gene is a piece of DNA which generates a protein that makes a chloride channel in epithelial cells. It is only when the variant of this gene is inherited that people have cystic fibrosis. In other words, we should be very careful to avoid associating a gene with the name of the disease caused by a variant of that gene.

One of the problems, then, that science journalists will have to face in the years ahead is how to get across a sense of the subtlety with which genes function in living things. It is a big intellectual task, which is obscured (to take a second example) when people announce, as they did in 1993, that the gene for male homosexuality has been found. It is incredible that it was put so blankly, yet this was in fact stated by the discoverers in the National Institutes of Health in Washington. We must watch out for the triumphalism of the geneticists — excited, as they quite properly are, by the immense importance of the discoveries now being made, by their significance for the long term and by their sheer intellectual interest.

*
* *

Discussion [2]

Durant: On the question of the role of the science journalist, I was trying to emphasize that a journalist is not de facto an educationalist. We need to recognize that these are distinct professions with distinct professional aims.

There may be an ambiguity in our paper. It was no part of what we wished to say that a growing minority of scientists support a dissident position on HIV and AIDS. (Indeed, we used the phrase "the overwhelming majority" to describe the majority consensus position on AIDS.) I was trying to refer to the appearance of dissent, several years ago, and eventually its manifestation to some journalists. It seems to have been journalists' growing awareness of the existence of dissent, however small-scale, that helped to trigger this particular episode. That is all that Mr Hansen and I wanted to say on the matter.

Wilkie: In terms of selling newspapers, a couple of years ago, the Americans announced they had discovered, as it were, rip-

---

2. Because it is short and comprises a heterogeneous collection of remarks and questions, the following discussion is presented as a continuous dialogue without subsections.

ples at the edge of the universe which were the seats of the inhomogeneity that gave rise to the galaxies and clusters of galaxies now observable. *The Independent* put that story as the front-page splash. This was one of the best-selling editions of *The Independent* on record. Science does sell newspapers in some circumstances.

A slightly different — and rather depressing — point: over the past year, the *ST* circulation has increased. Those who buy the *ST* are not moving against the paper, and its coverage of AIDS has done nothing to diminish its circulation.

The *ST* coverage indicates just how small the community of science journalists is in Britain. Essentially, the change of editorial line for the *ST* resulted from the views of two men, Neville Hodgkinson (science editor) and Andrew Neil (overall editor) of the paper: that is all it takes.

Finally, it may sound facetious, but it is important to say that the responses by the scientific community indicated by Professor Durant seemed to me woefully inadequate beside the point, and to misunderstand the social relations of science, newspapers and broader society. On occasion, I am asked to give talks to local meetings of the Institute of Physics or a similar organization. I have a little list of where journalists get their stories from. I go through the press officers, the press releases, and learned journals like *Nature*; then I come to the categories of "Hampstead dinner parties" and the "editor's wife". It is remarkable how often it filters down through the editorial hierarchy that the editor's wife has been shopping or having coffee or whatever with so-and-so who has said such-and-such — "...and is not that interesting?"

The other side of this is that editors of national newspapers do go out a lot, and they talk to a lot of people. But I would be interested to know just how often they meet scientists socially at these gatherings, and I would be prepared to bet that if the relevant people were attending the relevant dinner parties the *ST* AIDS coverage would never have got off the ground.

It would be worth asking when or how often in the past ten years the President of the Royal Society, for example, has invited the editor of a national newspaper to lunch. This sort of social contact between the scientific community, on the one hand, and the other institutions of society, on the other, seems to me to be one of the gulfs which the scientific community has failed to bridge. They are in a ghetto, talking amongst themselves, and not realizing that there is a different game that they have not even begun to play.

Shapiro: Excepting always the *ST* on AIDS, there is a danger that we may fall into the trap of shooting the messenger, an old habit that goes back to classical antiquity but is none the better for that. Take the homosexuality gene, so-called: where did that story come from? It came from a press release. Virtually every press story written in this country, as far as I could see, was done from the press release and not from the article. This was because the press release was made readily available by the National Institutes of Health. Do not shoot the press on that one.

Also, I am worried that the paper uses the ambivalence of the press as a criticism: the complaint is that the press is sometimes triumphalist and sometimes it expresses more worries than are justified about, say, genetic progress. Do we not all share this uncertainty? The Nuffield Council on Bioethics was founded at the instance of a lot of research scientists, medical professionals and science administrators because they were ambivalent. The ambivalence of the press so, far from being a matter for criticism, seems to me, merely to reflect the consensus of those who engage in this area.

Norton: I get the feeling that there is an undercurrent in this session that assumes that some scientists are dissatisfied with the coverage of science in the media. Is it, however, right or reasonable to expect science to be treated any differently? If we look at the press and media coverage of any sphere of current activity, whether foreign affairs, sport or domestic politics, none of it, except in very rare cases, complies with what a scientist might feel is appropriate — viz. thorough, objective and balanced coverage. It has to be recognized that there is an inevitable tendency to publish black or white and avoid the various uninteresting shades of grey in between. Since the public are exposed to all this tremendous variety in every other sphere, it can be assumed that they are fairly tolerant, and that a fair amount of damping goes on before they react to the latest story. It is probably better to get more exposure, and to suffer these vicissitudes of the press, than to shelter behind the laboratory door and get no coverage.

Hansen: There is a misconception in much discussion about the public understanding of science along the lines that science should have special treatment in media coverage. We do not agree, and are saying that some of the problems in the discussion about media coverage of science are precisely due to this misconception.

Andersen: I remind you that this is a conference on bioethics. I hope that, in this session, we can also draw in the problem of how the press deals with ethical questions. It is important to think about whether the press is contributing to public ethical debate, which is a part of the background against which parliamentarians decide ethical questions.

Hansen: We tried to indicate in our paper that the press does deal with ethical questions in coverage of the Human Genome Project and genetics more widely. We were not arguing that the press should not reflect the ambivalence that surrounds these issues, as was suggested by Mr Shapiro. Quite the contrary: we would agree that, of course, the press should reflect it. It is indeed reflected in the press that there are two contrasting discourses right from the outset of the Human Genome Project, which deal with, on the one hand, the tremendous promise of this kind of research and, on the other, the ethical and legal problems that are raised by it. One of the interesting things about that coverage is that, although ethical issues are mentioned time and again, they are mentioned in a ritualistic fashion. There is little in-depth discussion. I suspect that this is because the ethical debate itself is not very well developed. In addition, perhaps a problem for journalists is their lack of a set forum towards which to turn for information about the present state of the art in relation to ethical issues. The Nuffield Council on Bioethics is obviously an extremely important forum in this sense, but it may be that this debate can be moved on, only by having other centrally located fora towards which the media can turn. Finally, we should bear in mind that the media faithfully report on the activities of parliament — an institution which is assured of media coverage. Perhaps it is simply a case of providing more central fora for the discussion of ethical issues.

Durant: The tendency merely to mention in reportage that there are ethical problems, without in-depth discussion, points to the need for a higher level of ethical literacy; but it should not be assumed that the professional scientists or journalists are any better at knowing how to deal with ethical problems than anybody else.

Young: Professor Durant talked about the aim of the journalist. It is not the aim of the journalist that is important, but what he achieves. Even where his role (or purpose) is not educative, it is certainly informative — which, last, is a statement about the effect of his activities.

Can Professor Durant tell us anything about the different kinds of understanding of science, and the problems which have to be faced by the public, throughout Europe, which can be related in some way to the kind of information they are given through the public press? Does there exist in Europe a common underlying basis of public information about these topics?

Durant: As far as I am aware, there is no standard or uniform source of the best available current scientific information to which all journalists in Europe could turn. There is a variety of national agencies, offices of technology assessment, the Parliamentary Office of Science and Technology, and so on, which exist to try to provide information to parliaments and to users.

Young: I meant: how much is known about how well the public understands these particular issues? How successful have journalists throughout Europe been?

Durant: That is a big question. The best available information at European level is from the European Commission's eurobarometer surveys. There is also the media resource service of the CIBA Foundation, operating at a European level to improve the amount of scientific information available to journalists by enabling them to make contact with scientists.

Rodway: The British Medical Association (BMA) has an active public affairs division which acts as a source of information on medical ethics to the media from the perspective of practising doctors. Part of the problem in the United Kingdom is the fragmentation of the representation of medical ethics. The BMA has long been an advocate of a national medical ethics committee. The Nuffield Council on Bioethics is the nearest to this that we have.

Two further points. First, our views on the issue of doctors' involvement in inducements by drug companies to take part in drug trials were solicited by the *ST* Insight team; but we felt that we had been misrepresented. We wrote to the newspaper to put the record straight, only to find that our letter was itself edited. The media must operate properly in this area; they have enormous power, and therefore we expect equal responsibility from them.

Secondly, it should be borne in mind that researchers are constantly looking for sources of funds. The difficulty in getting work published in the scientific press, the publication bias, the practical difficulties, all mean that there will be increasing use of the media for this purpose.

Nairne: The theme of this session is the role of the media, but we have talked exclusively about newspapers; radio and television are often more appropriate in dealing with the ethical issues.

Robin Kent: There are some people in the BBC who make nothing but science programmes, but many of us are generalists. We may be working on one programme, and then suddenly we are working on a different programme, doing something about, *e.g.* genetics. Next week we may be on road transport policy. We often do start from a low base, and have to talk to people about the subject and make fools of ourselves. The more people can bear with us, and take a few minutes to explain to us the basics of, *e.g.*, the cystic fibrosis gene, the better it is.

Hansen: The claim that when there is distortion in the media, the problem may not be so much because the media are distorting information but that scientists are not communicating very well, leads on to the debate often heard in questions about the public understanding of science, namely, whether science journalists are sufficiently well trained, whether they should have a scientific background. Most science journalists do not come from a science background, but an arts or social science background. Science journalists would probably argue that it should stay that way because their important function is that of mediator. If they do not ask the basic questions about how things work in science, who should? In terms of communicating scientific information successfully and intelligibly to a lay public it is undoubtedly more important for journalists to be highly trained as journalists than to be highly trained in science.

Alastair Kent: I would like to interject into this discussion something of the perspective of those people who are the object of media stories about the genetic process: the families, the individuals who are directly affected by genetic conditions. In writing about complex issues, it is important to remember their impact on the expectations and hopes those families have for the future. We have to consider that the media — press, radio and television — are the mechanism by which most people who are directly affected by genetics find out what is going on. They see stories which reflect the exciting scientific advance, but also bring the realization that this is only the start.

Most families know that there is a huge gap between discovering the gene and developing treatment. Into this gap fall many of the ethical issues raised in earlier sessions. This is the gap where the negative outcomes of knowing about genetics arise as well as the positive options of developing treatment. I ask the media to recognize the excitement, but also the realities.

Greene: In 1993, the Research Trust for Metabolic Diseases was contacted by a lot of people because of the film, Lorenzo's Oil. For 11 years, we had been trying to get metabolic diseases on the agenda; suddenly we were in the limelight. Families were wanted for interviewing, and faxed information was required giving a potted history on the biochemistry of adrenoleukodystrophy (ALD). As a result, people were saying "ALD, Lorenzo's oil, myelin, myelin project, myelin sheath, multiple sclerosis (MS)... Lorenzo's oil helps people with MS!" Our office had to deal tragically with hundreds of people with MS who thought that Lorenzo's oil would be the answer to their prayers. It is important, then, that the people approached by the media are given time to give information accurately, so that it can be reported in a fair manner.

*
* *

Kennet : I want now to broaden the discussion to hear some news of what is done in other countries, and of what people from other countries think about what they hear is done in Britain over the whole field of genetic testing, without special reference to the Nuffield Report.

Kent: The Genetic Interest Group (GIG), with which I am involved, is a voluntary organization representing the interests of many single-disability genetic charities and support groups. Families who are affected by screening, and testing, say that an important factor in whether it has been a positive and successful experience is the extent to which they have been involved in the process — the extent to which they have understood what is being done, the reasons why, and the broader consequences it has.

Professor Brazier made some important comments on the legislative direction the issue of consent is taking, raising this notion of a fiduciary arrangement, an arrangement of trust. It seems to me there are great dangers with such an arrangement for the way in which people at risk of a genetic condition are involved in processes for which they give their consent. As I understand it, the basis of fiduciary consent involves the doctor (the professional) managing the information given to the patient so that the latter is able to reach a decision. The example quoted was of parent to child. I understand why people might think this an attractive concept, but I can hear the families in the membership of GIG saying "no". Good practice has moved away from the notion that "my doctor is my father" in many areas. I hope the legislators will not move in a direction in which that notional relationship is reinstated. Our legislators might wish to give some thought to the question how to ensure, in law, that people have access to all the information they need, and in a way that they can use it to make informed decisions for themselves whether or not to participate in screening, treatment and testing processes.

Kennet: There is a noticeable tendency in the United Kingdom to say this would be extremely difficult. We must ensure that anybody who faces a choice of this nature will have good counselling. We can write counselling into the Act of Parliament, or into the terms of reference of the study group or the controlling body.

Clarke: There are two crucial issues with the Duchenne muscular dystrophy newborn screening. First, the consent obtained from parents for newborn screening for an untreatable disorder has to be on quite a different basis from that for treatable conditions. Secondly, the importance is emphasized in the Nuffield Report both of pilot projects and also of evaluating novel programmes those where the long-term effects are not clear. Screening for Duchenne muscular dystrophy has been running now for approaching four years, but it is still too early for the full implications for the families identified to have become manifest. The social evaluation needs to be continued for a few more years before we are in a position to say whether this has been helpful to the families.

Holm: Consider population-wide screening, or screening of all pregnant women, even for a common genetic disease like cystic fibrosis: for it to be psychologically viable, I wonder whether it would not require the genetic literacy of the general public to reach a much higher level than at present. Otherwise, counselling would be prohibitive cost-wise.

Nairne: Paragraphs 8.4-8.7 of GSEI show that the Working Party and Council fully agree on the need for greater awareness and understanding of genetics and genetic processes. The point is very strongly made there.

Pembrey: Work in clinical genetics over 25 years has shown this: families very often do not want copper-bottom guarantees going as low as a 1 in 5,000, or less chance. It is sufficient if we can say their basic risk is something like a 1:500 chance, and very much lower risks can be offered for the vast majority. Even in the so-called intermediate situation, in which the mutation is found in one parent but not in the other, we are usually in a position to give them a figure they find reassuring. Families just want to know that they have done the responsible thing, got the information and taken it on board in making their decision. On the whole, they are reassured by being given risks of 1:300, or 1:500. These are small risks.

Shapiro: Professor Robert Williamson commented privately to the Nuffield Working Party, on the basis of the St Mary's London pilot study offering cystic fibrosis carrier screening to 10,000 individuals in North London, that his data indicated that counselling efforts could be concentrated on those who were identified as carriers of cystic fibrosis, rather than everyone entering a cystic fibrosis screening programme. This comment illustated the problems that we face when discussing resource allocation and counselling.

Super: With regard to concentrating the counselling on people who test positive, it is the right of anybody who has a test to have a letter stating what the result showed. This does not take an enormous amount of organization. Counselling is concentrated mainly on couples and people at big risk. Even when one person out of a couple is found positive, a letter is often sufficient, with an offer of intensive counselling for those who want it.

Kennet: Work carried out in France and by, I think, Professor Harper in Wales, showed that among groups of people who are well and truly counselled at all stages those who take a test and find they are negative cheer up, and those who take a test and find they are positive also cheer up. In other words, the counselling background being equal, it is the uncertainty that hurts more than the knowledge that you are on the wrong side of the line, which is very interesting.

Van Damme: Quite recently a law was adopted in Belgium according to which people must give whatever information they have on their genetic constitution when applying for life insurance. The Order of Medicine in Belgium, an extremely conservative institution, has forbidden any medical doctor to write genetic data on any form requested by a life insurance company.

Fluss: Dr van Damme knows the Belgian situation much better than I do, but I have in front of me a copy of a Belgian Law of 1992 on insurance contracts, and in Section 95, it specifically states that medical examinations must, under no circumstances, include genetic testing for determining the future state of health of the applicant for insurance. Section 6 lays down that genetic data may not be communicated.

Van Damme [interrupting]: I received the information very recently from a Belgian Parliamentarian who told me that such a Law has been adopted. The Order of Medicine has of course not reacted firmly against something that is non-existent. I read in their magazine that they were indeed reacting against this Law. I am not sure exactly when it was adopted[3].

Kennet: The situation revealed is of great parliamentary interest because, if you are both right, it is a very quick turn round by the Belgian Parliament (which is not impossible).

Dixon: Although this is a European meeting, it is not inappropriate to mention something of exceptional interest — the situation in China, with, as I understand it, explicit draft legislation which would use genetic screening for clear eugenic purposes[4].

It is also worthy of record that, by coincidence, a decision was taken at the International Congress of Genetics, in Birmingham, UK, in August 1993, that the next such gathering will be held in Beijing.

---

3. Dr Van Damme later confirmed that he had seen a proposal to amend the 1992 legislation, and that, when this legislation was indeed amended in March, 1994, Section 95 remained intact. Ed.
4. The national proposal in question was later put into abeyance, and laws remain provincial. Ed.

It has been said that not much is known about people's psychological reaction to having genetic information which is relevant to their future. What is the feasibility, and the desirability, of doing research into this, before particular tests become available? I have in mind things like alcohol dependency, for which there has been reported recently a putative gene. (I think the claims have been withdrawn, but none the less it is more likely than not that such genes will be identified. There will then be a situation in which people can have a test.) Say you are an alcoholic, you have the test and it is positive; will this make you feel you are predestined to develop alcohol dependency, or that it is not your fault[5]? Equally, if the test is negative, two correspondingly different reactions can be imagined.

Frontali: With regard to the psychological implications of knowing genetic information, in Italy the genetic counsellors usually play a kind of "game" before the test, and try out the worst scenario on people. The psychological implications of a positive test (which is of course the worst result) are explored with people. It is part of the way in which informed consent can be reached since it obliges individuals to face the psychological implications of the worst response.

Kennet: Winding up the session, I would like to thank Sir Patrick Nairne and Mrs Miles very much for giving us the opportunity to discuss the Nuffield Report, which is at the moment the principal document in the United Kingdom on this matter from both the political and the practical points of view.

---

5. Later in 1994, a case was reported in the US where a convicted murderer appealed against his conviction on the grounds that he was genetically disposed to murder, his evidence being the number of murderers in his family. Ed.

Legislation and regulation in Europe: experience and prospect

WAYLAND KENNET[1]

In this session, we turn our minds to what if anything Parliaments should do about the ethical and social consequences of the revolution in molecular biology.

To keep the subject within bounds, we have been using screening and testing as our example case. We have had two sessions exploring the ethics of screening, and one looking at how public information develops and operates. Now we are to think about public, and, in particular, parliamentary practice. In democracies, parliamentary debate is, or should be, prior to government practice: one of the roles of a parliament is to ensure that what the public is concerned about is faced and dealt with by the government.

First, what is it that's new in all this? What's worth holding a European conference about? Parliaments aren't new; ethics aren't new; testing and screening aren't new, even the European Community is no longer new. What is new is the revolution in molecular biology. Simply as a revolution, even that is not new: revolutions in science are giddyingly familiar, and have

---

1. Vice-President, the Parliamentary and Scientific Committee. Formerly British Government Minister and MEP.

become endemic in the last half century. But each one is different, and each one may or may not be of a nature which commands the attention of parliaments.

Revolutions in scientific understanding, in pure science, are generally not of this nature. The natural sciences describe, with ever greater precision and intricacy, whatever it is, out there, that appears to be the case.

But as soon as science can be applied, and is exploited in practice and technology, it often becomes a subject of ethical consideration. We judge it then no longer in terms of true or false, but in terms of good or bad, safe or risky. Thus, revolutions in applied science not only change the way we do things, they can also create new perceptions of present wrong and new expectations of future wrong, and these can be politically extremely compelling, and can in some societies and for a certain time, make some technological revolutions the principal subject matter of ethical consideration. They have to because the exploitation changes the relations between people, between societies, and between generations, and these are changes which will almost certainly generate in due course a demand for legislation or regulation.

Several revolutions in technology during the last two generations — new materials, electronics, computing, remote sensing — have created these perceptions in differing degrees. None so far has presented us with issues so compelling as the nuclear revolution. Nuclear fission and fusion, achieved and developed in secrecy for military purposes, were fairly soon felt virtually to embody the great dichotomy itself: use of the bombs became pure evil, the power stations and the diagnostics for a short time appeared as pure good. As a congeries of problems developed — military, political, economic, environmental — the evil side of the balance became the heavier. These changes changed the nature of relations between states and, when the effects of radioactive releases became clear, within states. The resulting demand for international regulation or legislation went unmet because there were, and still are, no supranational structures in existence which could legislate or regulate in the common interest. Nor were there even sufficient structures within states to foresee the problems, and to regulate in advance for the common interest. Just clearing up after the nuclear military, in both the United States and in the ex-Soviet Union, has become one of those mega-burdens to which we mostly shut our eyes.

What happened to the human race in that revolution was that we acquired the ability to wipe ourselves out: race-suicide had become possible. Parliaments came on the scene very late, and did not do a particularly good job when they did: state secrecy prevented them. But that time, neither commercial secrecy nor profit figured very large.

Now, let us turn to the revolution in molecular biology. First, the relationships of everyday life which will be changed by it, starting inwards and radiating out.

Personal self-knowledge will be changed.

So will relations between person and person: between lovers and other potential parents, and between them and their potential children; between natural and nurturing parents, and genetic and non-genetic children, between natural persons and manufactured cousins or even sibs, of whose existence the natural persons will sometimes be ignorant. And most recently between a person born of an egg taken from an aborted foetus and — well, and everybody else. As the Archbishop of York wrote last week: "What kind of a society is it which first kills its unwanted foetuses and then seeks to turn them into parents?"

Relations will also be changed between single persons and collective persons: between the individual and his or her employer, between the individual and the private sector insurance companies. And between the individual and the medical professions. Also between the individual and the community itself as the provider of health care and of national insurance; and as the maker of law, and as its enforcer. In short, between the citizen and the state.

Then, also between and among entire categories of persons: research and medicine, medicine and the state, medicine and industry, between research and finance, and medicine and finance and among industrial interests, especially pharmaceutical companies when they are taking out patents. At every interface, and they are of course far more than I have tallied, lives a layer, a complex folded layer, of ethical realities and puzzles that are, or can be, affected by what are, or appear to be, facts, newly ascertainable by screening.

Then there is, or soon will be, the fundamental argument, the argument about whether the present genetic foundations of the human race may be altered. By screening, germline therapy is made possible in this case or that, and many cases will soon make a class.

For Galton, eugenics was "the scientific study of the biological and social factors which improve or impair the inborn qualities of human beings". The word has now come most commonly to mean the ruthless and destructive use of the results of those studies: it has become a boo-word, and I suppose it has got to remain one.

But there will be slopes of all degrees of slipperiness in the forthcoming argument about germline therapy, and they are of very varying slipperiness. The simple seeming assertion, that, when on a slippery slope, one can stop whenever one likes, has one great weakness: the number of times people haven't. Galton himself in argument alone. The United States in practice in the 1920s, and indeed in the post war. Germany in the 1930s and 40s: the great exemplar which does, and should, dominate this debate.

Even now in China a law "on eugenics and health protection" is being considered. There are, the Chinese news agency says, "more than ten million disabled persons who could have been prevented through better controls". The controls proposed include prohibition of marriage, compulsory abortion, and compulsory sterilization. The draft does not deal with "artificial fertilization or test tube babies because the effects of these techniques have caused some disputes", and China has not yet decided whether to "adopt euthanasia to eliminate congenitally abnormal children, because the international community has not come to a decision on this issue".

It is against the background of a still living tradition that we have to face an argument that was faced too late in the nuclear revoution. It resides in the word-cluster "negligible", "no evidence" and surrounding homonyms: there isn't any real evidence that harm will or even might result but if any did, it would be negligible, therefore any responsibility for causing later harm now is negligible, and so on, in a escalation of reassurance, sometimes soporific, sometimes petulant. This was what was generally believed and said by governments in the 1950s about nuclear fall-out and waste.

There cannot be solid evidence in advance. The right course of action is one which takes account of that fact: the fact that "evidence" is not, and cannot be, available. Now the stakes are so high, the analysis of uncertainty in the assessment of the likely human and ecological results of scientific advance has become the most important part of that assessment.

The uncertainty analysis in the case of fallout from nuclear weapons tests was, we now know, wrong. Harm was caused, and the people who caused it are dead: mighty scientists in their ignominy, dead.

Looking into the double helix was a bit like looking into the nucleus of the atom. Shall we have learned? The revolution in molecular biology contains the seeds of the most potent perceived embodiment of the great dichotomy yet to have stressed human understanding. The nuclear revolution provided us with the means of species suicide which, with our usual attractive optimism, we have so far refrained from committing. The revolution in molecular biology seems likely to provide us with something it may be harder to resist, because it is not immediately clear whether we ought to resist it: and that is the means of refashioning our species.

Of course, if we were to contemplate doing that now, without any agreement on the direction in which we should, if at all, be refashioned, we should be committing an idiocy comparable to that of species suicide. Who are we to decide what we would like to be? A question surpassed in gravity only by the question: who are we to decide what we ought to be? And even if we had the right to do that, what about the physical uncertainty? Every time in this molecular biology revolution that a veil has been stripped from between us and understanding, another veil has appeared.

Don't we all want "better quality" births? How would it be if ever, some time in the far future, we were offered a chance of eliminating seasickness at will, or alcoholism? And what if we became sure, or what we considered sure enough, that germ-line procedures could, if universally applied, remove violence from among the modes of human action, and would have no bad side effects? What would be demanded of the power structures of that future time? Would this offer from science be one which democracy could refuse? What would the power structures be, anyhow?

The main completely new problem already with us is the forthcoming vast increase in the numbers of people involved: who may know, or may choose not to know, that their children in general, and then each in particular, have a given likelihood of getting some disease before birth, at birth, in childhood, or in middle age. There are no obvious maxims for these. How should "a society", whatever form that may take, cope at its own level with these new kinds of knowledge and these new tools?

There are also large-scale social problems, that derive from the unprecedented scale of the new possibilities: how many of us will be deemed truly healthy when we are all being screened for everything? If it is the case that one in three of us will die of cancer, in middle age or before, will this group of us become a sub-class? There will be a knowable proportion of people who are going to develop that, or some other lethal or semi-lethal condition at some point: will they become the designated unemployable, in an economy where unemployment is finally recognized and admitted to be a tool of policy? The latest budget in the United Kingdom puts the burden of sickness benefit onto employing firms. And will not tax-payers want to be sure that those for whose training they are paying, as, say, doctors or architects or soldiers, will live beyond twenty five years?

In the face of the foreseeable and early changes in a large number of social relationships, and of the many remote possibilities which are hard to foresee, it seemed a good idea to find out what the national parliaments of the European Union were already doing about it.

You have before you notes of the law now in existence in the countries of the European Union on testing and screening for HIV and for genetic disease, provided by the World Health Organization, to whom our thanks are due for this work[2].

We also decided to find out how our own parliaments made their minds up what to do, and what structures and procedures they used. So we set up our study of national Parliaments in the European Union, the first results of which are among your papers. The work was hard to confine within the limits: it showed a healthy tendency to turn into a sample-slice study in the morphology of democracy itself.

Five parliaments are covered, and the remaining seven will be covered after this conference, when we shall have had the benefit of your comments on the work done so far. The five authors of these papers have followed more or less closely a series of questions which was put to them: that is what gives their common pattern to the papers. I will not try to summarize the results: they reveal more similarities than dissimilarities, in my opinion.

This is not surprising. Each of our parliaments arose, or at least took its modern form, for the same reason. Mostly they were, and still are, expressions of the need, increasingly felt between the seventeenth and nineteenth centuries, for an ever increasing proportion of the peoples to have a say in the making of law, until in the last two generations that has become virtually everybody. Their growth has also been part of, and symbolic of the national independence of our countries. If you look at the pictures of our national parliament houses which are on the cover of the paper I have referred to (where they are didactically left unnamed) you will see ideograms of democracy and of national distinctness. With few exceptions they also speak of pride in nationhood and in the national stability which democracy is supposed to ensure, and in fact so often does.

Though there are many resemblances, there are differences among them. Perhaps the most interesting is the existence or non-existence of a national ethics council.

There is a French slogan: from Ethics to Law. In a sense, there is no other route to law than through ethics: no other reason to make new law than somebody's perception that it would be right to make it, and wrong to leave it unmade. And this applies to all law, even the most humdrum: somebody, according to some lights, however dim, is convinced that a deserving section of mankind will be happier or better off if the change is made. No perception of rectifiable wrong, no new law. But though ethics may be the only route to law, it does not follow that law is the only thing ethics can lead to. It can lead to professional regulation and all points downwards: government advice, professional advice, and so on.

There is, in human nature, a scale of different possible reactions to the slogan: from ethics to law. At one extreme is the temperament which feels, if it's wrong, we must legislate at once. Let us forbid it in the Penal Code, or at least write it into the Civil Code, and if we can't do either of those, then let us outlaw it in some other code or body of law, such as the Public Health Code. The British think that is the French way.

At the other extreme is the temperament which feels: if it's wrong, let us educate everybody to know that it is wrong, and that will surely solve the problem. At the very most, let us hope the professionals will regulate it in their own codes of practice; medical, nursing and so on. Above all, no new law. The French think that is the British way.

Where a national ethics council exists, it will not necessarily affect the position on that scale its parliament adopts. But what it will do is bring the skills of moral philosophy regularly to bear on legislation. Given the present status of ethics itself in some of our countries, that is an urgent task. Moral philosophy is still emerging, in some countries, from a half century of neglect. So much so that there are many in parliaments and in governments who believe either that ethics does not exist, or that it is something quite other than what it is. In either case they are left at the mercy of their individual and often unexamined apprehensions of common sense.

Examples of the mistake that ethics does not exist are before us every day in this country. It is as though the whole thread of western wisdom from the pre-Socratics on had been judged inconvenient, perhaps as standing in the way of other goals. These goals were first, in the 1930s, scientific progress, which was supposed to be real in a way that ethics could not be; and more recently the pursuit of wealth in economic freedom, which alone is supposed to constitute a real good. If that is one's scale of values, then of course the only way of deriving policy from judgment is by deep excision of the offending matter of ethics from personal consciousness.

As an example of a mistaken belief that ethics is other than it is, I would offer the following from a recent report on the ethical regulation of certain clinical procedures commissioned by the British Government: "Ethics are the moral convictions of thoughtful, conscientious and informed people [deriving] from a compound of natural philosophy and religion..." The text goes on to say that natural philosophy and religion are intuitive, and that "rules and duties" are derived from "utilitarian principles". This is a way of saying that ethics are fuzzy beliefs entertained by good-natured people. One cannot say this if one has any acquaintance with the idea that ethics is a part of philosophy in general, and that philosophy is, in the words of R.G. Collingwood "organized and systematic thought directed towards the discovery of truths concerning a definite subject-matter". That sort of thought is quite difficult, but there are people who can do it.

National ethics councils are a convenient method of bringing such people to the fore. If properly constituted, they will have a membership which is able to juxtapose conflicting insights, wring out the elements of pseudo-conflict, and agree on a submission or opinion which brings out the true conflicts in measured and comprehensible terms. Committees tackling ethical or ethico-legal problems without any moral philosopher on board, and in this country they are the rule not the exception, are like committees designing bridges without an engineer.

There is another scale revealed in our study of parliaments: that between relying exclusively on chosen learned bodies and on the other hand consulting the people directly on actual issues as they arise. Ethics is an exact study, a philosophical discipline, yes. But many of the schools it contains and the conclusions they reach correspond quite closely with what many people thought already. It is extremely useful to elicit their ethical opinions from the uninstructed. In this field Denmark is, among the European Union countries, undoubtedly the most experienced. The Danish consensus conference system is simple in purpose and highly sophisticated in execution. All our countries and their parliaments would be the better for learning from it.

There is also the scale between restrictive national climates of opinion and permissive ones: meaning restrictive and permissive about interventions in the processes of nature, and of the Tao. This scale is more experience-linked, and consequently each generation will be to some extent determined by what has happened in the preceding couple of generations.

Germany's place on this scale comes from the experienced horrors of genetic intervention. It is one of the few fixed things in the moral firmament of Europe. Survey after survey shows up, in bioethics, the Spanish drive towards maximum freedom, and the Swedish preference for sober restrictions: direct reactions to the deeply-anchored preconceptions of a few decades ago. This might lead one to conclude that even if it were possible to achieve harmonization in our laws, and regulations about bioethics within the Union at a particular moment, yet it might prove difficult to preserve it, at least at first, as old national elasticities were still working themselves out.

But do we want harmonization at all, or even a single regime? We deliberately did not put a picture of the European Parliament on the cover of our document, in case it should distract the mind from the disparities we have now. It seems clear that we must know and understand these disparities better than we do before we can begin to approach the question of harmonization.

Certain questions, though, may already suggest themselves as a framework for discussion. I will suggest two.

1. Are the following among the advantages of a plurality of regimes:

— the natural diversity of humanity?
— the greater importance of smaller exclusive groups feeling at home with their laws than of larger inclusive ones feeling at home with theirs?

— the possibility of pleasing more people in total by diverse local regimes than could be pleased by a single Union-wide one?
— the existence of factors likely to cause opinion to vary over time in a different way from country to country?

2. And are the following among the advantages of a single regime:

— the convenience of pharmaceutical companies developing the relevant substances and treatments, and the theoretically lower prices which could be achieved?
— a single regulatory approach to licensing arrangements with countries outside Europe?
— the preclusion of "medical tourism" in the fields concerned, that is, going to a country with a more relaxed attitude towards the treatment you want and buying it there, which you can in any case only do if you are rather well off?
— freeing resources, including ingenuity, for action to bring the benefits of the revolution in molecular biology to the Third World?

In some areas, it is impossible to judge in advance how things will — or should — work out: how, under subsidiarity, will national health and national insurance schemes operate? What about pharmaceutical firms' profit rates where a monopoly product is one of enormous importance to the whole community, including the poor world?

What about the growing impact of commercial interests on parliaments? The "health and insurance industries" in the United States have poured $150 million into congressmen's private pockets in the last decade to stop Congress changing the existing US health system[2]. They have been completely successful. That is beginning to come our way too.

How will decisions be taken about who may benefit from a vastly expensive process for which there is unlimited demand, not only in the rich world, but in the poor? We will begin with

---

2. *International Herald Tribune,* 14-12-93, p. 2.

the heroic treatment of individuals, probably individual children, whose situation will be irresistibly appealing and touching, but behind whom are other children, in their millions.

All these things will give rise to their own extremely complicated debates, and combined with the debates which will continue below on each national level, and above on the Pan-European and on the World levels, it does seem likely we should not hurry.

Yet how can we not hurry, given the huge breadth of the scientific programmes and their rushing acceleration, epitomized by the human genome programmes? The discrepancy between the democratic tortoise and the scientific/industrial hare is potentially tragic. We need consensus conferencing, and professionally constituted national ethics committees, and probably everything in between as well.

The role of parliaments

WAYLAND KENNET[1], LARS KLUVER[2]

The Danish experience of Consensus Conferences

Consensus Conferences have been held regularly in Denmark since 1987. Through them, the Danish Board of Technology and the Danish Parliament become aware of the lay-response to technological and scientific issues which involve ethical and political questions. Some subjects which have been covered are:

— gene technology,
— agriculture in industry,
— food irradiation,
— mapping of the human genome,
— genetically manipulated animals,
— traffic and the environment,
— childlessness.

In 1994 there will be Consensus Conferences on:

— integrated agriculture,

---

1. Vice-President, the Parliamentary and Scientific Committee. Formerly British Government Minister and MEP.
2. Head of secretariat, the Danish Board of Technology.

— SMART cards as identity cards,
— virtual reality.

The conference involves two panels, the most important of which is the Citizens' Panel. It consists of fifteen lay people attracted by advertisements in local newspapers. The panel personnel changes entirely from conference to conference. Usually, between 100 and 250 people apply to take part. In choosing this panel we do not claim to be representative. A mixed panel is chosen on the basis of demographic data, such as age, sex, region in which they live, level of education, and occupation. There is a narrow concept of what is meant by "layman". The layman must have no connection with the profession under discussion.

The job of the Citizens' Panel is to draw up the main questions for the conference: to set the agenda. At the conference, the members of the panel listen a great deal, and they write the final document which is discussed on the last day.

The second panel is the Expert Panel. There were fifteen experts at the Consensus Conference on the Human Genome which I shall take as an example. Between ten and eighteen experts may attend, depending on the subject and on how many experts it requires. The concept of an expert is broad, and anybody who is able to contribute with insight can be regarded as an expert: thus it can include people from grass-root and environmental organizations. Patients may be experts if they can tell other people something they did not know previously and which is relevant for the subject. The role of an expert is to present matters from the expert viewpoint and answer questions raised by members of the Citizens' Panel.

The procedure of a typical consensus conference is as follows:

(a) Advertisement/selection of the Citizens' Panel. This is done by the secretariat, but there is a planning group of experts, members of the Board, and parliamentarians if the conference is being held in co-operation with Parliament. This planning group approves the suggestions we make about the panel, and considers all the applications.

(b) First weekend. The conference is held over two weekends. During the first, the Citizens' Panel discusses the relevant values. Perhaps we play a game with them in the course of which they pick values they think are important. In the example I am presenting, they were given education in basic genetics by a high school teacher. We do not want to use the time of the actual conference on simple biological matters.

(c) Second weekend. On the second weekend, the Citizens' Panel draws up the main questions for the conference.

(d) The planning group selects the experts. The planning group suggests appointments to the Expert Panel. The lay panel accepts and approves these. This is done by the lay panel between the two weekends if possible, when there is an idea of what the main questions will be.

(e) During the above phases, the members of the Citizens' Panel are given various materials. We ask them if they want much or a little to read — and they always say they want a lot.

(f) The conference usually lasts three days: the first day is tough. The experts give presentations, answering the questions asked by the lay panel. At the end of the day, the lay panel has to go on working, to consider what kinds of questions and areas have been evaded, or not yet been covered. The second day is a half-day, and on that day the Citizens' Panel puts these further questions, and the experts try to answer them. The Citizens' Panel then writes a final document during the evening — and the night. (I do not remember any conference when we have stopped before 6 am. We are now beginning to have a day off in between because it is too tough.) On the last day, which is usually a half-day, the final document is presented and discussed at the conference. There is also a press conference in addition to the presentation.

The final document reflects: the knowledge and (if there is one) the consensus of the experts; the opinions of, and disputes between the experts; the values of lay people; the fact that the experts do not agree on some things — a conclusion regularly seen which is a problem. We must have more discussions on these disagreements, and the scientific community must work on them.

Parliament usually takes up some of the results. Following the consensus conference on the human genome in 1989, for example, there is now a commission in Parliament working on the regulation of gene testing, pensions, employment and insurance. The press responded actively with headlines; there were two transmissions on television news and a lot of radio coverage. This conference was held in the Parliament building, and some of the Members of Parliament "attended" (*i.e.* came in and out).

This methodology is successful in terms both of political life and of discussion in the press. It should not be seen itself as part of the media because people taking part in the conference are usually selected in some way. The discussions afterwards in Parliament, in the newspapers and the press, are the important media for this.

*
* *

Discussion

Vaughan: As a parliamentarian, how effective do you find these consensus conferences, Mrs Husmark? Also, who selects the topics for the conferences?

Husmark: I agree with Mr Kluver that if it is to be a democratic process, it is extremely important that there is no bias in the selection of the lay people, and that the experts come from a broad area (so far the Danish Board of Technology has succeeded in achieving this); but I do not agree that it is only the "club" that takes part in Consensus Conferences. There is a good link between the professionals and lay people.

The Board of Technology selects the topics, in close association with the Parliament and the press, and having regard for what society needs.

Shapiro: How much does a conference cost?

Kluver: Depending upon the aims — and on such things as travel expenses — between 35,000 and 50,000 pounds. The work of a commission, or social scientific research project, costs about the same.

Young: Does this procedure mean that the work of parliamentary committees is shorter and easier, so that money on parliamentary funding can be saved while it is spent on the conferences?

Husmark: The committee work in the Danish Parliament is not on one topic, but on running the legislation. The planning process is so long that the conferences do not usually have a significant influence; but the knowledge that emerges from these consensus conferences can be used to plan legislation, and this can be done in a more competent way.

Reiter-Theil: How are the experts selected? Indeed, what is an expert? What, *e.g.*, would be competence in medical ethics? There can be experts of different kinds, professional experts and moral experts. Can you comment on this?

Kluver: We work with what we call "counter-expertise". We try to have experts from both sides of an issue; and as I said, the concept of an expert is broadly construed: we have had chairmen of patients' organizations, environmental activists, patients and industrialists.

Durant: I am interested in the emphasis placed on the conference itself as an opportunity for parliamentarians to see the process of dialogue and exploration going on. I had assumed that the principal value of the conference to those not involved would be through the ensuing public debate and the final report; but you seem to be saying that holding the conference in, or near, the Parliament buildings is an important asset.

Kluver: It is important, because being inside the conference room, and getting the "feel" of proceedings, differs from merely reading about the results in the newspapers.

Husmark: Attending the conferences also provides the opportunity of dialogue there with the audience: we meet people who are very much interested in the topic under discussion, and then we take things further in the parliamentary process, the press, or wherever we work.

Greene: What is the period between placing the advertisements to the final report being issued?

Kluver: The Board works on the conference for about 18 months to define the issue. The project itself takes nearly six months.

Iglesias: Does the majority of the people in Denmark think this method is fostering democracy and is good; or do only those who are interested in the topic put their names forward and discuss the matter — with the rest of the population not caring very much?

Kluver: I think the results of the conferences are disseminating into society. The method itself is not very much communicated, so it is not surprising that the man in the street does not know how a Consensus Conference is organized.

Sandberg: Consensus Conferences on medical problems have been tried in Norway, but Norway has never been willing to take the risk of having a lay panel: they have two expert panels — one witnessing and one writing the report.

Could Mr Kluver describe an issue which is not suitable for a consensus conference?

Kluver: Air pollution. Consensus conferences are not a good method if we want very stringent and systematic results; they are good where there is a basis of knowledge and opinion in society. The conference on air pollution failed because we wanted a plan of action, which is too systematic a task for a lay panel meeting only on two weekends and working overnight.

Nairne: I had the impression that the timing of the conferences was linked in some way to the parliamentary programme. Parliament is often under pressure to act swiftly, but public opinion takes time to mature, and it can change. I would have thought that the question of timing is important.

Secondly, I was fascinated to learn that there are equal numbers of people on the Expert and Lay Panels. How often has it emerged that the Citizens' Panel rejects the advice of the experts? Or, in practice, do the experts' views tend to dominate?

Kluver: We usually advertise for suitable issues in professional magazines and our own magazine. Letters are sent annually to about 1,000 addresses in Denmark asking for ideas for issues, and usually 100-150 suggestions are received. The Board ends up with about 20 issues which the secretariat then describes and assesses for suitability. The Board then decides which to pursue.

Turning to your other question, on the last day of the conference we go through each page of the report and the experts can correct factual claims that are incorrect; opinions cannot be corrected by them, though. I do not think their views dominate.

Van Hoeck: Would you say that the homogeneity of Danish society, and the size of Denmark, are elements which explain the success of consensus conferences?

Kluver: I have no examples of conferences being held in mixed societies, but I think this method could be used in any society.

Andersen: A consensus conference on traffic and the environment proposed that we raise — I think, double — the price of petrol. A poll carried out in the population at the same time would have given a different answer. I think we should be a little wary of the representative value of the conclusions of the Lay Panel.

Kluver: This result really "hit" the press. In fact this one part of a plan in which the money from the high price of petrol would be used to lower the registration fee on the new and environmentally sound cars. The idea was that, in the long run, these cars would be so efficient that their running costs would be the same, but there would be less pollution. This idea did not come through to the press.

The conclusions of the Lay Panel are not representative: this is an informed panel, more informed than the general public. I think this is valuable, because it shows what the population would say if the education and public debate were greater.

Botros: I am sceptical about the notion of an ethical expert. If there is a dispute between two scientists, it is quite natural to throw that back to the scientists to come to some agreement. If there is a dispute between two moral philosophers, surely that is a matter for the members themselves to dispute. Do you recognize that distinction? You said, also, that there was quite a lot of ethical reflection implicit in the Lay Panel's report. I wonder whether the Panel could explicitly defend its judgements insofar as those involved ethics.

Kluver: The Lay Panel are not trying to compromise, or to argue in favour of one person, or another person, but trying to express their own feelings, their own ideas about how things should be. They do this after listening to the experts. We cannot claim to have anything but implicit ethical judgements from such people.

Botros: My point is that your view on a scientific matter could be justified by pointing to the experts; this cannot be done with ethics.

Durant: The value of a small number of lay people giving their view in this way is an interesting issue. The notion of public opinion is slippery. Measurement of public opinion, even on matters of high public salience (*e.g.* which party should be in government) is notoriously unreliable. When it comes to science and technology, where public awareness and involvement is still lower, the value of taking general random sample surveys seems to be much more doubtful. The special value of the consensus conference is to demonstrate what a group of people who have worked through an issue might then think about it. The process the lay people go through is appropriate if we want to know something about considered opinion on a subject.

Dixon: Are attempts made to balance the panel — on, say, age? If consensus conferences were conducted in countries where there are contrasting religious views, would you wish to move towards a balanced sample — to include people from particular viewpoints?

Kluver: The answer to the second question is No, not usually. Our usual aim is to find people who are open-minded, and if an applicant has an extremely solid opinion about the issue, this person cannot contribute anything to the process. However, with the conference on childlessness, an attempt was made to have one person who favoured adoption, one who favoured the exploitation of scientific techniques, one who just accepted childlessness, and so on. A balance was sought.

Norton: The Danish Technology Board and the Parliamentary Office of Science and Technology (POST) are co-members of the European Parliamentary Technology Assessment Association. Sir Gerard Vaughan will be familiar with the US Office of Technology Assessment (OTA), set up in 1972 to provide Congress with help in dealing with scientific and technical issues. So a spectrum of organizations has been set up to help parliaments to deal with these issues. The Bristish approach is focused on the decision-making and debating process within Parliament, seeking to inform that debate in an objective manner. It is more closely tied into the parliamentary business than is the approach of the Danish Technology Board.

The European Parliamentary Technology Assessment Association recently held a meeting on bioethics which brought together the activities of all the various groups in that general field. We heard from:

— the Danish Board of Technology on the recent consensus conference on infertility treatment;
— the French on their large project on bioethics which is so crucial to the current debate before the French Parliament on a number of Bills in that area; and
— the British and the German approach, discussing the Nuffield Council type of approach, for example, to screening.

Vaughan: Although funded by our Parliament POST is totally independent of the Executive, just as the American OTA is totally independent of their Executive. There was a time when the American OTA began to get a bit involved with its Executive, and almost immediately the effectiveness of its reports dwindled.

Short presentations by relevant intergovernmental organizations

S.S. FLUSS[1], G. KUTUKDJIAN[2], A. ISOLA[3], J. ELIZALDE[4]

World Health Organization, Mr S.S. Fluss

I will focus upon WHO's Health Legislation Unit (HLE). Key activities of this unit are: (1) The HLE journal, *International Digest of Health Legislation*, is used in parliaments as a source of information on legislation derived from primary sources; (2) HLE has a library on bioethics, and on health and environmental law; (3) databases have been developed, some of which deal with genetics, human experimentation and transplantation; (4) surveys of legislation have been carried out; (5) HLE has interns, mostly from the USA and Canada; and (6) the unit has also been involved in human rights activities.

Since its first appearance in 1983, AIDS legislation has been monitored in such countries as the Channel Islands, the UK, the Russian Federation, Uzbekistan, Grenada, both of the Koreas, the former GDR and the US. We are able to handle about 30 languages. We rely exclusively on original texts, and

---
1. Secretary, WHO Working Group on Human Rights. Formerly Chief of WHO Health Legislation Unit.
2. United Nations Educational, Scientific and Cultural Organization, UNESCO.
3. Directorate of Legal Affairs, Council of Europe.
4. Head of Unit E.5. of DG XII, European Commission.

prefer to do our own translations to ensure that the versions are unofficial but in line with contemporary terminology on both sides of the Atlantic.

In Europe, in the early period (*i.e.* 1983-1984), information with a bearing on AIDS was not shared adequately between parliaments, between governments, between government departments, between the universities, and between public health officials. If we look, for instance, at the origins of the blood scandal in France and elsewhere, it is apparent that certain mistakes could perhaps have been averted by an improved flow of information. This is where the Unit is important. It provides the basis for contacts within the European Union but also outside it. One day perhaps we can bring in bodies such as the US Congress where there is a great interest in bioethics and AIDS issues; and why not also Canada, and Central and Eastern European countries which are not part of the European Community?

We have developed legislative databases and some publications. The publications have been done commercially. About three weeks ago, *Legislative Responses to Organ Transplantation* was published, a copy of which has already been sent to the Council of Europe. (Mrs Annick Isola, from the Council of Europe, has said that it is very helpful to their work on organ transplantation.) We are working on another book, *Legislative Responses to Ethical Issues in Human Experimentation*, and a second edition of *Legislative Responses to AIDS* (1989) is being contemplated in the light of developments since its publication.

A sister organization of WHO, the Council for International Organizations of Medical Sciences (representing the medical disciplines and the national medical associations), is holding a series of conferences within the context of a dialogue on health policy, ethics and human values. The next conference in this series (Ixtapo, Mexico) will focus on, inter alia, major international trends in bioethics and health policy ethics.

Finally, I offer an extract of a speech made very recently by the Director-General of WHO, Dr Hiroshi Nakajima, at the opening of the 93rd session of WHO's Executive Board, which indicates that, in the coming months and years, WHO may well play a more active role in bioethics.

"My intention is to push for WHO's intensive involvement in the fields of both human rights and biomedical ethics. With its global membership, long-standing experience of standard setting and specific technical expertise, WHO is uniquely equipped to facilitate reflection, exchange of data and experiences and consultation at the international level. As one distinguished member of this Executive Board very aptly put it, WHO should be the health conscience of humankind" (Geneva, 17-1-94).

UNESCO, Mr G. Kutukdjian

The subjects of screening for HIV, and for genetic disorders, and bioethics in general, need to be addressed at international level. To give a recent example from the world conference on human rights in Vienna in June 1993 (which is not necessarily verbatim): "A reflection at the global level should be matched by action, both normative and educational, in a broad sense. The urgency of the issues and the high stakes should not prevent exchange of ideas and clarification of concepts which are crucial steps in standard-setting activities and harmonization of laws and regulations."

It is within this framework that the Director-General of UNESCO in 1992 created an International Bioethics Committee, chaired by Noelle Lenoir, Member of the French Conseil Constitutionnel. In November 1993, the general conference of UNESCO approved the creation of this committee and gave it a mandate to prepare an international normative instrument for the protection of the human genome. In preparing this international instrument, the Committee identified four areas for priority in 1994-95:

(1) The state of knowledge in genetics. In this area, the sharing by the North, South, East and West, of knowledge, in particular of the mapping of the human genome, is essential. The economic implications of this knowledge are equally essential, as are the ethical issues involved in research and the responsibility of the researchers.

(2) Genetic testing and screening questions, such as: Who decides on testing or screening? For which illnesses or disorders should there be testing or screening? Which body will be the depository of genetic information, which might acquire significant size and meaning over generations and lead to possible misuses, including control measures over individuals or groups?

(3) Genetics of populations, demography and development. In this area, we ask: How can the misuse of genetic material of ethnic groups be prevented, as well as discrimination against them or, for that matter, population control policies? How can economic claims to genetic material be tackled when that material is used for commercial purposes?

(4) New treatments generated by genetic engineering, such as gene therapy, medicines or vaccines, which may be produced for diseases such as malaria.

The reports produced on these topics will converge on the preparation of the international instrument for the protection of the human genome. The committee has outlined principles, very much line with the opinions expressed during this conference, and grounded in the rights and liberties enshrined in the universal declaration of human rights and related international instruments. These are:

— the freedom of research,
— the responsibility of the research community,
— human identity and dignity,
— the protection of private and family life,
— the autonomy of the individual, and
— solidarity between individuals, communities and nations.

Finally, I wish to indicate that the Committee stressed the importance of training, education and information to accompany any standard-setting action. Public, informed debate to raise the level of awareness must be encouraged so as to fill the gaps between the research community, decision-makers and the public at large. This is an unavoidable democratic challenge. To succeed, legislative action must be founded on a clear understanding of the issues and choices to be made.

The Council of Europe, Dr. A. Isola

One basic goal for the Council of Europe (CE) is the protection of human rights; hence the Council has been active in the field of bioethics. The CE's interest here covers testing for genetic diseases, and for HIV. With regard to the latter, the Committee of Ministers of the CE — conscious of ethical issues deriving from the need to balance individual and collective rights and duties — adopted the recommendation R89/14: *The Ethical Issues of HIV Infection in Health Care and Social Settings*. This enumerates principles countries should consider when dealing with HIV. Voluntary testing was recommended since, when integrated with counselling, it is the most effective approach from the public health point of view, and the most acceptable ethically and legally. Of course, voluntary testing must be supported by information campaigns, respect for confidentiality, and a policy of non-discrimination.

Progress in genetics is one of the most promising ways to reduce human suffering, but it also raises fears. This observation was the starting point of the second symposium on bioethics of the CE in December 1993, which focused on ethics and human genetics. One session here was devoted to confidentiality issues arising from genetic testing. The problems aired in this session included the conflict between the right to privacy and the fact that knowledge about genetic disease in one family member may have important implications for the health of other family members. The other issue was the risk of discrimination, if genetic information were to be used by third parties, especially employers and insurance companies. According to a number of speakers, the disclosure of information to insurers would have serious disadvantages both for the individual and for society. In 1992 the Committee of Ministers adopted a recommendation on genetic testing and screening for health care purposes. This recalled basic principles in this field:

— the requirement to obtain free and informed consent,
— the non-compulsory nature of the tests,
— the need for appropriate counselling and support.

The recommendation also stated that insurers should not have the right to require genetic testing, or to enquire about the results of previously performed tests as a precondition of the conclusion or modification of an insurance contract.

This conclusion will be carefully considered by the Steering Committee on Bioethics of the CE, which is currently preparing a draft bioethics convention on the protection of human rights and the dignity of the human being with regard to the application of biology and medicine. This will be a framework convention containing general principles; and it will be complemented by protocols. Two protocols are currently being prepared, on organ transplantation and medical research. Preparation of a protocol on the protection of the embryo will start soon. Since it will be a framework convention containing general principles, national legislators will be required to implement these principles when they become parties to the convention.

So far, the draft convention contains two articles on genetic testing and screening. The effect of the first draft article is to restrict the use of tests which are predictive of genetic diseases to health care purposes or scientific research. The second article deals with the communication of results of such testing. The rule is that such communication should be limited to the health field. It will however be possible for national legislators to permit the communication of test-results outside the health field when there is an overriding interest.

In conclusion, a few words on parliaments: the CE aims to set out standards for the protection of human rights in the field of bioethics. Although the texts are aimed at governments, national parliaments have a great role to play. Indeed, the parliamentary assembly of the CE comprises MPs of each member state. There is no doubt that parliaments play a great role in protecting human rights. It is with the help of parliaments that we shall ensure that the bioethics convention is not a technocratic text but a truly democratic one.

The European Commission, Dr. J. Elizalde

I work for DG XII, as head of a unit working on the ethical and legal aspects of life sciences. The work on the regulation side of screening is done by DG V. I will explain how the European Commission deals with bioethics, and with screening, from the research side.

Bioethics is mainly a "subsidiarity" field: the Commission does not act where national parliaments and governments are already active. But on research, the Commission has taken a proactive role to some of the new technologies. For example, a conference was organized in Mainz in 1988 on human embryos and research.

We have pushed, through a reluctant European Parliament (EP), a programme of research on human genome analysis. The EP is a budgetary authority, so, we need its approval.

Here we can add to the list of legislation from HLE[5], *Human Genome Analysis* (the Council Decision), and the useful *Ethical, Social and Legal Aspects* report.

5. *Laws, Regulations, and Other Legal Instruments on Screening/Testing (Genetic and HIV) Adopted Under the Auspices of the European Community and the Council of Europe, and by Member States of the European Community,* which was distributed to delegates at the conference.

We have a committee on the ethics of biotechnology which reports directly to the President of the Commission. We are responding beyond genetics to the whole field of medical ethics, and are funding teams throughout Europe.

The EP displays a great interest in the ethics of biotechnology, prenatal diagnosis and the ethical aspects of patent law (matters beyond research), but there is no European code of legislation on bioethics (one is being developed in the Council of Europe, the right forum, because it is a consensus platform. The Council of Europe works by co-operation between governments and institutions in each country; the European Union works through integration, which is probably not the right method for bioethics).

There are three bioethical principles governing research which are part of the programme now almost adopted after consideration by our ministers:

1. Research on germline gene therapy, and therapy itself, should not be continued.

2. Linked to the media debate, is the ban on cloning the nuclear substitution, of course, of human cloning.

3. Encouragement to develop alternative methods to the use of animals in research.

Invited contribution

COLIN CAMPBELL [1]

I will describe the work of the Human Fertilization and Embryology Authority (HFEA) which provides independent regulation in an area in which, in the United Kingdom, matters are controversial and the issues sensitive, and where both the treatments on offer and the risks involved go beyond the doctor-patient relationship. The HFEA was established by statute to license and regulate clinics that carry out donor insemination, in vitro fertilization and human embryo research. Parliament passed legislation to ensure nationwide oversight of two main areas: (1) the creation or use of human embryos outside the body; and (2) the use of donated genetic material — although the work of the HFEA also covers the diagnosis in the embryo of genetically inherited disease prior to being transferred to the woman.

In regulating treatments and research, the HFEA has to consider:

— the interests of the patients;
— the interests of the prospective children;
— the public view on the research and treatment;
— Parliament's wishes; and

---

1. Chairman of the Human Fertilisation and Embryology Authority, United Kingdom.

— matters affecting safety, efficacy, ethics and the desirability of the treatments being on offer in the first place.

The HFEA represents one model for dealing with ethical issues within a legal framework. One of our tasks is to ensure that people in the United Kingdom are properly informed about and involved in discussing the ethical implications of new developments. At the same time, Parliament gave the HFEA relevant powers to curtail work, so that scientific developments are properly controlled in this country.

Parliament insisted that the chairman and deputy chairman of the HFEA should be laymen to ensure that there is representation of public opinion. Scientists and clinicians are included in the membership of the Authority to advise them. Our statute prohibits sorts of work to which Parliament is opposed, such as the creation of hybrids (mixing animals and humans). As to existing treatments and new developments, the HFEA is required to consider what is "necessary or desirable", flexible words whose implications may change over time.

We have drafted a code of practice, giving advice about how conduct should be promoted and what treatment should be provided. All centres are also inspected to make sure that we know what is going on under Parliament's name. One of the roles of the HFEA is to consult the public and to inform them of what is going on. We consult the profession, patients and the public. In 1993, a document was published asking the public whether sex selection should be allowed not only on medical grounds but also on social grounds, and overwhelmingly the public said No. Regarding the possibility of being able to take ovarian tissue from an aborted foetus, mature the eggs, store and use them, the HFEA recently published a document asking the public whether they want this sort of work. Ten days after this document was issued 5,000 copies had been requested by the public, so it is clearly a matter of concern.

In an area of this sort it seems to me that the role and limits of an independent regulator such as the HFEA are tested. The prospect of using eggs from foetuses was not envisaged by Parliament when it passed the legislation: MPs may wish to look afresh at issues that are potentially of great significance and, if Parliament wishes to do so, it will. This does not undermine the status, or the independence, of the Authority; for we can describe the issues for Parliament and for the public, promote debate and consult on Parliament's behalf, advise in the chambers of Westminster, and bring our own experience of scrutinizing ethical issues. And, of course, if there is to be excited debate about the use of ovarian tissue, the Authority can meanwhile reassure the public that such work is not going on, and that there is no current intention to license it. Vitally, the HFEA has to give advice to the Secretary of State and lay a report before Parliament every year. Parliamentarians have an annual opportunity to check whether things are developing as they wish.

As a model for establishing an interface between law and ethics, the HFEA is a positive and useful example, in that it establishes a framework, but does not close down debate; watches the progress of new developments, but brings in national, social and ethical dimensions; receives, and balances, the views of scientists with those of patients, ethicists, philosophers, churchmen, laymen and others; and can advise Parliament of issues that need to be discussed and determined again within Parliament.

*
* *

Discussion

Vaughan: The British Parliament is extremely pleased with the way in which the HFEA has been functioning. It has enormously reduced anxieties in this field. British MPs have received many letters on these issues.

Husmark: The parliamentary committee for the Danish Council of Ethics is debating the aspects of biomedicine discussed by Sir Colin Campbell. This should lead to the setting up of a board, not identical to the HFEA, which will look at new activities in the area of human fertilization before they are put into action.

There will be an amendment of a law made 18 months ago which, as it emerged, concerned only experiments on human fertilization and not treatments, leaving it to the doctors to define whether something is experimental or a treatment.

Van Hoeck: Not much has been said about the role of the European Parliament (EP) which plays an increasingly important role in the European Community. Amendments put forward on two occasions by the EP have had a direct bearing on the problems discussed during this conference. The EP has continuously asked for an increase in Community funds for research on AIDS; they have been increased, following this action by Parliament. Secondly, the inclusion of a research area in the biomedical programme on biomedical ethics is the consequence of an amendment put forward and adopted by the EP. The Commission proposal did not cover this area of research; the EP added it, and this was accepted by the Council.

Now the Maastricht treaty has been adopted, the EP will become more important, as regards research, since Parliament will have the power of veto over a Council common position. This means that Parliament will be able to co-decide with Council in the future.

As regards national parliaments, they sometimes feel that it is useful to interact directly with Commission officials. Most of them do it occasionally, but three parliaments do so more often than the others. The parliament that does it most frequently is the British Parliament. The British Parliament, its committees and select committees, often call on Commission officials to provide written or oral evidence — or even send delegations to Brussels to discuss matters with the Commission. The two other parliaments which also do this are the German and Danish Parliaments. Others do so less frequently.

Rodota: In Italy, we have not had parliamentary discussion of reproductive technology and genetics, because the majority party in Parliament, the Christian Democrats, is strongly opposed to any legislation in this field. They maintain that to legislate in this area means legitimizing, in reproductive technology, what has already been condemned by the Roman Catholic Church.

In the last few weeks, there has been discussion in Europe of the pregnancies in older women both in England and in Italy. The man at the centre of this is Italian. This development was possible in Italy because there are no rules regulating the centres working in this area.

Walton of Detchant: In Britain, the House of Commons (HC) is the final legislative assembly. The House of Lords (HL) acts in many ways as a revising chamber. It can amend legislation coming up from the HC, but it is ultimately up to the HC to decide whether to accept those amendments. The HL has no final authority.

The HL has a mixed membership of hereditary and life peers, now more than 300 of the latter. Vitally, there are 270 cross-bench peers, not affiliated to any political party. Some of the life peers have previously been Cabinet Ministers in the HC; others have come from industry or from the professions.

Legislation, not least in the bioethics field, may be introduced first in the Lords, before being considered by the Commons. This was the case with the Human Fertilization and Embryology Bill, now an Act, about which we have heard today.

The HC and the HL appoint Select Committees, usually of not more than 10-16 people, to investigate important issues. Their reports are debated, and may provoke legislation.

I served on a Subcommittee of the Select Committee on Biotechnology. We spent a great deal of time visiting European centres and centres outside Europe, learning about biotechnology. The report, which was debated in November 1993, recommended that the present European Commission directives on biotechnology are excessively restrictive, and overemphasize the potential dangers of the release of genetically modified organisms in the medical, scientific and agricultural fields. A number of recommendations were made which will be considered by Parliament to see whether any submission should be made to the European Commission.

A final point relating to professional self-regulation: Can this be extended on the European scale? It has been in medicine. I was formerly the President of the General Medical Council, the self-regulatory authority concerned with the regulation of medicine in the UK, which gives ethical advice to the medical profession. I served on the Conference des Ordres de Medecins, the European-wide body of such regulatory authorities which also, like the Council of Europe, UNESCO, and WHO, gives ethical advice on matters of scientific and medical importance. I firmly believe that there are certain issues of ethical principle where European consensus can and must be achieved. I am nevertheless equally confident that subsidiarity in this and other fields must be maintained, because certain such issues can properly be dealt with, only at the local and national level.

Dunstan: As regards legislation and regulation, there is a lesson to be learned by analogy with the control of innovative embryology and *in vitro* fertilization. The success of the HFEA derives from six years' experience of regulation by a voluntary licencing authority. This authority won the confidence of the relevant professions (scientific and medical) and accustomed them to inspection, regulation and licencing. This was done entirely by consent. In doing this, the real problems to be addressed were learned — which were not always those perceived by the public. Local ethics committees were set up to act as local watch-dogs on practice and on relations with a central ethics committee. I believe the voluntary authority had the confidence of the public, and it was never severely criticized from outside. This gathering of experience moreover enabled a quick and clean passage of the Bill creating the HFEA through both Houses of Parliament. I plead now that experiment to gain experience in co-operative regulation precede legislation.

Walton of Detchant: The Government has established a voluntary committee to supervise work in the United Kingdom on gene therapy. In a similar way, this committee may ultimately become established by law as a statutory authority.

Shapiro: There is an important difference within Europe between societies where professional self-regulation has been the norm in medical ethics, and societies which need to legislate. The French need to legislate, whereas Germany, the Netherlands, the Scandinavian countries, and Britain have been used to self-regulation. In comparing parliamentary systems, we must look not just at the particular parliament, but at its relations to other law- and rule-making bodies.

Dalla Vorgia: In Greece, we have recently passed a law providing for the establishment of a national ethics committee, and also for ethics committees in hospitals, and private clinics.

Kennet: Are the latter committees research ethics committees or also clinical ethics committees?

Dalla Vorgia: The law does not exactly specify; a ministerial decision will state clearly and in detail the tasks of these committees.

Giesen: I am less optimistic about professional self-regulation in the field of bioethics. For the good of society, and to have an adequate representation of all sorts of interests and values, it is better to entrust the regulation of research to legislators.

Society should be in command, and the best way to do this in a democracy is through its elected members in parliament.

Walton of Detchant: Professional self-regulation can work properly only if it is subject to informed lay opinion and advice. This, by the way, was also Ralf Dahrendorf's view. Further, it is a principle of British society that the common law is better than statutory law.

Vaughan: In the United Kingdom, we move increasingly to statute law; it was for this reason that we insisted in Parliament on having a lay chairman of the HFEA.

Iglesias: As a professional moral philosopher, I find a great reluctance by scientific groups to reflect on ethics and to formulate those ethical principles which, the scientists themselves think, should guide their profession, and to take responsibility for those guiding principles. Medical people do — and have a duty to do — this. But over all, there is very little attempt to take responsibility for the ethical principles governing the professions, by the professionals. It may be important in journalism, medicine and science to have small international conferences where professionals establish the ethical principles lying behind their activities. When they have agreed these, communication can begin with parliaments and other bodies.

Andersen: What ethicists have to offer are intellectual tools. They can clarify the moral thoughts which people have. Ethicists cannot solve any of the problems in a substantial sense, but they can ask about consistency, cogency, and so on.

Kennet: In the course of discussions on the Bill which set up the HFEA a few years ago, Dr Sophie Botros gave seminars at the House of Lords for Parliamentarians and their staff on the rights and wrongs of this contentious Bill. When legislators — and indeed political animals at any level — face each other, one side says we ought to do this, and the other side says we ought to do the opposite, and they take a vote without further analysis. This is how politics is normally conducted. It can be extremely valuable to have a moral philosopher present at an early stage who is accorded sufficient status to be allowed to say to both sides "Let us go into the question of *why* you think we ought to do this".

Rodota: I am worried that public opinion and legislative bodies may react in such a way that we don't pass from ethics to law, but from scandal to law — legislating following pressure of public opinion generated by a reflex emotional process.

Kutukdjian: In France, those concerned with public information wonder what strategy to adopt. Television programmes dealing with scientific matters have been unsuccessful; and journalists wonder whether to organize round-tables and public debates at local level to bring together scientists, parliamentarians, and the public, or whether to forget the adult population and target young people.

Hutton: In the voluntary sector we want the chance and the time to examine an issue of this kind from a whole range of possible perspectives: ethical, religious, and that of public health. Yet, we inevitably find ourselves scrambling behind the process of Parliament, not knowing where we stand, or when something is going to be debated. This militates against calm, collected, and rational consideration of the issues described by Mr Kluver.

The future

General discussion

Kennet: The purpose of this session is to collect ideas for the future. This is the first of a series of five conferences, so it would be interesting to have ideas that might be discussed at the remaining meetings about things that could be done in any country of the European Union — or in one country and adopted in others. (The Danish networking is an obvious example.)

What else could the European Commission do? Dr Elizalde has told us that bioethics is to remain very much on their agenda; we have heard the same from the Council of Europe, WHO and UNESCO. What might these organizations do?

Elizalde: The Commission seeks a co-ordinating role at European level. The task is not always easy. To give an example: there is a draft Directive on the confidentiality of databases which has implications for medicine, particularly for epidemiology. It would be wrong to make it obligatory to have consent for every transmission of data. If this were agreed, epidemiology at the European level, using automated information, would become impossible.

Also, may I mention that our DG V Commissioner for Employment, Industrial Relations and Social Affairs, Mr Flynn, is planning a meeting of experts on medically assisted reproduction. We want to organize one or two workshops on this subject.

Fluss: The Cellule de Législation Comparée of the French Senate regularly publishes reports on existing legislation in countries of the Community and countries such as the United State of America and Australia. As far as I am aware, access to these reports is, by no means, limited to the members of the French Senate. It may also be of interest to mention that the Office of Technology Assessment (OTA) of the US Congress published a report that examined policy-making in bioethics in different countries just five months ago. Studies of this kind, covering the countries of the Community and with somewhat more detail than was possible in the OTA report, would certainly be of use.

WHO is associated with an initiative, undertaken with the support of the Ethics Committee of the Human Genome Organization, designed to produce an annual yearbook tentatively entitled Genetics, Ethics, Law and Society. A month ago a planning meeting was held in Washington, DC. I am convinced the editors, Professor Alex Capron (University of Southern California) and Bartha Knoppers (University of Montreal) would welcome contributions from specialists and the Institutions of the Community.

At a number of universities in France, including several in the Paris area and at least one in Lyon, courses in bioethics are taught in departments of external studies, in such a way that physicians, lawyers, nurses, prison administrators and government officials, etc. are in a position to attend. Generally this entails approximately one day a week over a period of three months. I believe that this is a very valuable approach.

Finally, developing countries clearly welcome access to the literature of bioethics. Obviously their funds are very short, so if there is any way in which the Community could assist the flow of bioethics literature in such languages as English, French, and Spanish, to universities, government departments, and non-governmental organizations in developing countries, this would seem to me to be a very useful initiative.

Reiter-Theil: This type of conference would have been easier if preceded by specific research, so that we could then discuss the results of that research at the conference. For the conferences which follow, I hope that the research which cannot be conducted within the project group can be substituted by the use of other research resources.

Dixon: Scientific societies and major international scientific congresses ought to do a good deal more than they currently do to involve the public in their affairs. This would enable the public to see what is going on in science, and the scientists to become more acquainted with people's concerns. The International Congress of Genetics (held five-yearly, most recently in 1994 in Birmingham, UK) recently decided to have a fully developed public awareness programme within what would otherwise have been a purely scholarly congress. The organizers allowed the public into sessions specially convened for them, every evening and for the final day. A booklet, called *Genetics and the Understanding of Life*, was also prepared and presented to those attending the public affairs programme. In spite of the misgivings felt by one or two people on the Executive Committee, this was an enormous success, with over 400 people at every session and high quality discussion. There was a further penumbra, if you like, of awareness through the media, locally, nationally, and indeed internationally.

The programme was not cheap, but the cost was justified. The Birmingham programme, funded by the Gatsby Charitable Foundation, cost 25,000 pounds. I would contrast that with the last European Biotechnology Congress (1993), where there was neither public awareness nor public involvement, and where there was no press involvement either. Efforts are being made to persuade those responsible for the next Congress to ensure that the press and public are catered properly for. I would encourage anyone who has an influence on gatherings of this sort to try to raise the funds and bring in the public.

Alastair Kent: The discussion at this conference would have been enhanced by a more overt presence of two groups which are not represented here very highly: the beneficiaries of medical progress — those who have genetic conditions, or are HIV-positive, their families and carers; and, with quite different values, which we ignore at our peril, the people who want to make money out of what we have been discussing — the commercial sector. Most people in the first group are without the means to attend a gathering of this sort without financial support. Such support must be budgeted for, if the voice of the "user" is to be heard in the debate.

Kennet: With regard to the pharmaceutical industry, I made every effort to obtain representation, but did not succeed. We have been fortunate in having plenty of first-rate carers here, and I was relying somewhat on the carers to say whether there should also be sufferers present. In fact, there have been sufferers among us, but they did not figure as such — they were here for — as it were — some other skill that they have.

Nairne: There is a pressing need for continuing communication between all those who are directly and responsibly concerned with bioethics. I believe it would be of value to hold a conference annually to keep us up-to-date on developments.

Part two

BIOETHICAL INFORMATION IN THE NATIONAL PARLIAMENTS OF THE EUROPEAN UNION

Introduction

WAYLAND KENNET

The papers which follow describe how information about the progress and potentialities of the revolution in human microbiology, and its actual and potential ethical and social effects, is at present acquired and handled in the national Parliaments of the European Union. Screening for HIV and for genetic disease, the subjects of the January 1994 conference, are accorded particular attention as examples which to varying degrees hold good for the entire field in different parliaments. Five of these twelve papers were completed before the London Conference, and the remaining seven afterwards, taking into account the lessons learned from the first five and from the conference itself.

They were all based on an initial outline which had been elaborated in co-operation with the intended authors of the first five papers. Each paper was itself usually worked out in advance at a meeting with the author(s). The outline was devised to catch as much as possible of what went on in the various parliaments.

The approaches and assumptions of the various papers differ one from another, as was to be expected and welcomed. The differences of presentation are themselves informative about the parliament of each country, and the resemblances are informative about that shared practice of democracy which is the basis of the European Union.

The larger countries' parliaments have the most comprehensive sources of information. Some parliaments rely heavily on extra-parliamentary sources; some on government-provided information; some, for reasons which will be obvious — church-state relations, for instance — have not addressed certain bioethical questions at all.

The conference organizers and the editors of this book most cordially thank the writers for the heavy task they undertook.

Bioethics and the Belgian Parliament

GEORGES BINAME [1]

The constitutional and political framework

To understand the Belgian situation in the field of bioethics, certain characteristics should be kept in mind:

The constitutional framework

Since May 1993, Belgium's Constitution has begun with these words: "Belgium is a federal State which is made up of communities and of regions."

There are three communities: the French-speaking community, the Flemish-speaking community and the German-speaking community. In the same way, there are three regions: the Walloon, the Flemish, and that of Brussels.

Belgium also consists of four linguistic regions: the French, the Dutch, the German, and the bilingual region of Brussels.

Each level has its own government, parliamentary assembly, and powers. If we take the example of AIDS, preventive measures are taken by the communities, health care is provided by

---

1. President, the Belgian Association of Bioethics.

the federal State, and the hospital infrastructure by the regions. Thus the Communities concerned with prevention may develop different policies, and questions of ethics associated with AIDS will be similarly sliced; hence, the need to develop collaboration between the different institutions (federal, regional, community) which may include co-operation agreements.

These institutional complexities are the price Belgium has to pay to overcome its various tensions, conflicts, and divergent interests in a peaceful and pragmatic manner.

The political framework

Since 1918 Belgium has been run, with few exceptions, by coalition governments, whose programmes bear witness to the Belgians' capacity for compromise.

Moreover, the judeo-christian morality prevails in our country, but presents a philosophical cleavage between two strands of institutions: catholic and lay. Moreover, differences of sensibility, mentality, and traditions of thought distinguish the French-speaking and the Dutch-speaking parts of the country in a marked philosophical pluralism. These differences prevent neither dialogue nor the pursuit of common positions, but they are strong enough to give quite specific orientations to such ethical committees as may be created.

The questions of bioethics fit awkwardly within the consensus of governments: they divide the parties, debilitate Governments, create shifting majorities, and can indeed trigger a constitutional crisis, such as the refusal of King Baudouin to sign the law on abortion.

The Pact of Government of 9 March 1992 states that for the matters it does not cover, the "parties of the majority have agreed to abide by the classical rule within a majority, namely that such matters are treated on the basis of a consensus within the government, and among the groups of the majority in the Parliament". Implicitly, this language aims at bioethical questions.

It is in this constitutional and political context that in Belgium bioethics is evolving.

The channels of information

Internal channels

1. Parliamentary control over the action of the executive is exerted by means of:

— written and oral questions;
— interpellations in committee or in plenary session;
— interventions in the course of the examination of budgets and of Government bills.

Parliamentarians currently use these procedures to get informed and to control Government action. The greater part of information obtained in that way is published in the form of parliamentary documents.

2. Parliamentary initiative

— *The creation of a capacity for Technology Assessment:* On 8 December 1992, the federal Parliament organized through the Committees of Public Health, of the Environment, and of Agriculture of both Houses, a "biotechnology day" when addresses were given by a dozen experts. The meeting had the great merit of establishing a dialogue between the scientific world and the political world. As was said at that time: "some scientists expressed themselves in a comprehensible manner, and some parliamentarians were disposed to listen to them". At the end of the day, participants unanimously and clearly expressed the wish to pursue the dialogue.

In November 1993, two proposals were laid in the Chamber of Representatives. The first was to create an "Advisory Committee on scientific and technological questions". The second was to create "a mixed Committee for the Evaluation of scientific and technological choices within the Belgian Parliament".

Though their philosophy, purpose, and institutional framework are very similar, the two projects differ fundamentally concerning composition, organization, function, logistic support and finance. These two projects are being currently examined by the Economic Commission of the Chamber.

— *Organization of hearings, "information days" and seminars.* For instance, a Biotechnology Day in 1992.

— *Creation of study groups within the parliamentary groups* whenever this is felt necessary.

— *The library of Parliament:* data bases, press service, loan of books, a bioethics documentation service.

— *University collaboration:* each parliamentary group is assisted by a group of university collaborators responsible for preparing parliamentary briefs.

External channels

1. National

Federal Government initiatives

— The organization of conferences: In May 1987, on the initiative of the Minister of Public Health, a conference on "Bioethics in the 1990s" was organized, gathering Belgian specialists and researchers. The principal conclusion was a wish to set up a "permanent structure for study and discussion". In May 1987, in the context of the Council of Europe, the Minister of Justice organized an international conference which examined the juridical aspects of artificial human procreation. The need to set up a National Ethical Committee was among the conclusions. In December 1993, when Belgium held the Presidency of the Council of Ministers of the European Union, the Minister of Public Health organized a conference on Organ Transplants in Europe.

— The creation of a Bioethical Consultative Committee: Since 1985, successive coalition governments have announced their intention to endow Belgium, like France, with a national consultative body on bioethics; but it was only in 1993 that the National Consultative Bioethics Committee was actually founded. This committee is a traditional one in many ways, but it has some peculiarities which allow it to fit into the Belgian institutional landscape.

• Traditional aspects: The Committee will provide both advice and information: it will give advice on its own initiative, or on request from persons or authorities entitled to, on problems raised by research and on the application of its results in the fields of biology, medicine, and health, whether these problems concern the individual, social groups, or the whole society. These problems are examined under their ethical, social, and juridical aspects, including in particular those respecting the rights of Man. The Committee will also: inform the public, the Government, the Parliament and the community councils; create and maintain a document and information centre; organize a conference every other year on ethical problems in the life sciences and in health. The Committee will consist of 35 members chosen for their expertise, their experience and their interest in ethical issues. A balance of representation among the different ideological and philosophical tendencies will be sought; so will a balance between men and women.

• Peculiarities: In Belgium, bioethics "exploded" among the different political levels, each with its own powers, hence the need for the representatives of the Federal State, the regions, and the communities, to co-operate within the Bioethics Committee. Linguistic parity has to be maintained between Flemish and French speakers.

Various other sources of information

— the research departments of the political Parties;
— the various conferences and publications of academic and other associations and centres for the study of bioethics;
— the quarterly report on the epidemiology of AIDS in Belgium, produced by the Institute of Hygiene and Epidemiology;

— the publications of the AIDS Prevention Agency of the French Community;

— individual contacts with the Churches, the Universities, and firms;

— the 1989-1991 report of the "Belgian Register for Assisted Procreation".

2. International

— There is a Belgian representation at the:

• Parliamentary Assembly of the Council of Europe. This institution is currently examining a project for a "European Convention on Bioethics";

• Interparliamentary Union and the International Assembly of French Language Parliamentarians (AIPLF).

— Association with the European Science Summit organized by the European Parliament on 14-15 October 1993 in Brussels.

— The work of the Parliamentary Committees has included:

• In January 1991, a delegation of the Committee on Public Health and the Environment to the Institut Pasteur in Paris, and a meeting with Professor François Gros, a biologist.

• In February 1991, a delegation of the Committee on the Economy and Scientific Policy to Heidelberg, including a visit to the European Molecular Biology Laboratory.

Belgian legislation in the field of bioethics

Government initiatives

1. At the federal level

Blood:

— Framework Law of 7 February 1961 concerning therapeutic substances of human origin. Three principles: exclusion of commercial transactions, protection of the donor, and therapeutic purpose.

— An Arrêté Royal (secondary legislation) of 10 November 1971 on the procurement, the preparation, and the delivery of therapeutic blood substances of human origin.

— Law relating to blood and derivatives of blood of human origin (Document 1229/1-93/94). This completes and reinforces the law of 7 February 1961 and the Arrêté Royal of 10 November 1971, taking into account the assimilation of several European directives into Belgian law and the drama of the haemophiliacs contaminated with HIV. Although in Belgium only a small percentage of haemophiliacs were contaminated with HIV through blood transfusions containing factor VIII, it has been the object of permanent attention from the safety section of the transfusion system.

Organ transplants: The first transplant in the world of an organ from one living person to another — a kidney — took place 3 on June 1963 at Louvain. It caused a storm of indignation, but marked a turning point in the history of organ transplants, and such operations were soon accepted by the international scientific community and the world in general. A law of 13 June 1986 tends to encourage transplantation, on the basis of he following principles:

— presumption of solidarity,
— freedom from charge: the human body is outside commerce,
— anonymity for both donor and recipient,
— therapeutic purpose,
— free, informed and conituously revocable consent for the removal of an organ from a living donor.

Artificial insemination: Article 38 of the Law of 31 March 1987 "modifying certain legal dispositions concerning affiliation" provides that, where paternity is contested, disaffiliation "may not be granted if the husband has consented to artificial insemination or to another act to secure procreation, except if the conception of the child cannot be the consequence".

Human genetics: The development of human genetics is partly dealt with by the "Higher Council of Human Genetics", which was founded in 1973. and in part through the information, consultation and research activities of the Genetic Advice Centres attached to university hospitals, which have been subsidized by French and Dutch Communities since 1989. A paragraph has been inserted in clause 5 of the Law of 25 June 1992 on insurance, which covers disclosure to the insurer. The new paragraph constitutes a limitation of the general principle of the obligation to disclose known risks to the insurer. It is headed: "Genetic data may not be communicated." An Arrêté Royal of 14 december 1987 regulates Centres of Human Genetics. The eight which already existed were made part of the hospital programme.

2. At the community level

To improve the success of the fight against AIDS, the Council of the French Community created a co-ordinating *Agency for the Prevention of AIDS* by its decree of 16 April 1991. The Agency's role is to:

— undertake, organize or encourage initiatives for the prevention of AIDS;
— co-ordinate such initiatives;
— collect documentation in the appropriate disciplines;
— establish contacts with public and private institutions working in this field and respond to their requests;
— represent the French Community at appropriate scientific meetings;
— advise the Executive on requests for subsidies.

The Agency for the Prevention of AIDS is directly under the authority of the Minister of Health of the French Community. Beside its functions of direction, co-ordination, management, accountancy, secretariat, etc, the Agency has at its disposal resources for planning and for programme evaluation. The persons concerned will help the services responsible for the prevention of AIDS to set up their programmes in a coherent manner.

The Agency will collaborate with international, national and community institutions, and with the schools of public health. It will also regularly enter into contact with outside consultants, whether Belgian or international (for example consultants in public health, in health economics, in communication...).

The Agency will regularly publish information on the programmes it has undertaken, as well as recommendations issued by the Scientific & Ethical Council.

The Decree of 16 April 1991 created a Scientific and Ethical Council within the Ministry to ensure that all preventive action is based on scientific rigour, dialogue and consensus. This Council has two sections:

— The Scientific Committee, the purpose of which is to advise the Minister, at his request or on its own initiative, on the priorities for control of the epidemic. This Committee is composed of scientists and researchers specializing in the prevention of AIDS.

— The Ethical Committee, which is to advise the Minister — at his request or on its own initiative — on any ethical or juridical aspect of the fight against AIDS. This Committee, representing various ideological and philosophical tendencies, is composed of jurists, philosophers, specialists in bioethics...

Parliamentary initiatives

The law of 3 April 1990 concerning abortion: Article 2 establishes that no offence is committed when a pregnant woman, whose condition places her in a distressful situation, has requested a doctor to terminate her pregnancy. This termination must take place before the end of the twelfth week. It must moreover take place in favourable conditions (medical infrastructure, psychological counselling and information).

The law of 13 August 1990 created a National Commission of Evaluation on the application of regulations about the termination of pregnancy. Every two years, the Commission submits to Parliament: (1) a statistical report; (2) a report detailing and evaluating the application of the law; (3) If need be, recommendations for a possible legislative initiative and/or other measures which might contribute to reducing the number of terminations of pregnancy, and to improving the guidance and the welcome available to women in distress. Information gathered by the Commission is confidential and may in no case be communicated to others, even the judiciary. The National Evaluation Commission has so far brought out two reports, covering the period from 1 October 1992 to 31 December 1993, and has stated that this is still too short a period to allow any recommendations for legal reform.

Bioethical information in the Danish Parliament

BO ANDREASSEN RIX [1]

In the last ten years, the discussion of bioethical issues arising from new biological technologies has intensified dramatically in Denmark, as it has in many other countries in the world. Already in 1984, some members of the Danish Parliament (Folketinget) argued (in a debate) for legislation to ban medical research in genetic manipulation and further advances in fetal diagnosis. In the eighties, the Ministry of Interior set up a Committee to discuss social, cultural and ethical aspects of the new reproductive technologies, and genetic testing and screening. Following the recommendations of its report "The Price of the Future" in 1984, the Danish Parliament passed a law in 1987 establishing the Danish Council of Ethics, which is now very active in the assessment of the ethical impacts of developments in biomedicine. Following a discussion of biotechnology, in 1986 the Danish Parliament established the Danish Board of Technology, which has arranged meetings and consensus-conferences *(see below)* in the field of technology assessment.

In the late eighties and early nineties, most assessments of cultural, social and ethical impacts of new medical technologies such as genetic testing and screening have been initiated

---

1. From the Danish Council of Ethics.

by the Danish Council of Ethics, and, to a lesser extent, by the Danish Board of Technology, often in opposition to the interests and points of view of the authorities. Thus, by establishing bodies such as the Danish Council of Ethics, the Danish Parliament has deliberately created the basis for independent advice on the ethical questions involved in new medical technologies, independent of the Government as represented by the ministries, and of interests groups, both religious and professional groups (*e.g.* doctors). The Council of Ethics and the Board of Technology are funded by the Danish Parliament, and could thus be seen as public watchdogs and independent sources of information to the Parliament.

The Council of Ethics and the Board of Technology spend about 10 m DKR (1.3 m ECU) a year on workshops and meetings, reports and other publications, as well as funding analysis of the ethical, social, legal and cultural aspects of new biological technologies. The Council of Ethics has a staff of 5 and the Board of Technology a staff of 13. The Board of Technology rely on contractors to do reports on technology assessment, while the Council of Ethics writes its own reports and, to a lesser extent, contracts out.

Information to parliament about genetic testing and genetic screening

The Danish Council of Ethics

Following several discussions in the Danish Parliament, the Council of Ethics was established in 1988. It has 17 members of whom 8 are appointed by the Minister of Health and 9 by the permanent parliamentary committee which follows the work of the Council *(see below)*. The operation of the Council is independent of the Ministry of Health and other administrative bodies, and it reports directly to Parliament. This special status, independent of Government and administrative interests, gives the Council more credibility. Under its terms of reference, the Council makes proposals to the Minister of Health on specific bioethical subjects such as the protection of human embryos and fetuses, prenatal genetic testing, and the registration and use of information about genetic diseases and genetic traits. The Council also advises the health authorities on general bioethical questions, informs the public, and initiates public debate on bioethical issues.

The Danish Council of Ethics has already published reports on most of the tasks defined in the law which set it up. It has also adopted an information policy to initiate public debate on the issues before it. These debates bring forward different points of view in order to obtain a dialogue between opposing views, and through them, the public influences the Parliament's discussions.

The Danish Council of Ethics has released about 40 reports, books, booklets, research papers etc. on issues such as the criterion of death, the protection of human embryos and fetuses, prenatal diagnosis, mapping of the human genome, genetic testing, genetic screening and allocation of medical resources. It has also arranged major hearings on issues such as the protection of human embryos, prenatal genetic testing and genetic screening, and some of the hearings have been held on the premises of the Parliament in order to make it easy for members of Parliament to participate. The very intense effort by the Council of Ethics to inform the general public about bioethical issues and to generate a public debate promotes open discussion, because different interest groups such as doctors, religious groups, and patient interest organizations take part. Thus the debate makes it possible for politicians to be confronted with different arguments, to make their own statements, and to follow the reactions to these statements among the public.

The Parliament's Committee on the Council of Ethics has 9 members, reflecting the political balance of Parliament. The Committee appoints the members of the Danish Council of Ethics, and it follows the work of the Council. Most members of the Committee on the Council of Ethics are also members of the Health Committee of Parliament, as some of the work is closely related. The Committee on the Council of Ethics receives very few communications from interest groups concerning bioethical problems: the primary official source of information is the Council of Ethics itself, which is often approached by such groups. The Council of Ethics sends copies of its reports and recommendations to the Committee on the Council of Ethics, as well as to the Health Committee of Parliament. The yearly report of the Council of Ethics contains a section on the work of the Council as well as recommendations from the Council on bioethical issues it has discussed during the past year. This yearly report is sent to all members of Parliament. Reports from the Council of Ethics are also sent to the Minister of Health and other relevant persons such as researchers and administrators in the Civil Service.

Following the release of a new report with recommendations, the Council of Ethics holds a joint meeting with the parliamentary Committee on the Council to discuss the issues, and the recommendations put forward by the Council. There are also regular meetings between the Council and the Committee to discuss the work of the Council, and future projects. The members of the Committee and other MP's are invited to participate in the public hearings held by the Council of Ethics on bioethical issues. Members of the Committee on the Council of Ethics are also invited to participate in the Council's visits to research centers and hospitals with the purpose of getting a close and realistic impression of the techniques involved, and having an opportunity to discuss bioethical issues with the researchers in their own environment.

The members of the Committee as MPs participate in a number of political and other meetings all over the country and the contacts made at these meetings are a valuable source of information to the politicians on bioethical as well as other issues. The press is also considered an important source of information on biomedical issues, especially concerning single issues of interest. Often MPs take part in the media debate by writing letters to the editor or giving interviews. General debates on bioethical issues such as genetic screening and testing only seldom take place in Parliament, because of the heavy workload from economic and other big issues.

Interactions between the Danish Council of Ethics and Parliament in the field of genetic testing, genetic screening and related issues

In 1988, when the Commission of the EEC presented its research programme "Predictive Medicine" to promote human genome research in Europe, the Danish Council of Ethics submitted a report to the Minister of Health. It concluded that the mapping of genetic susceptibility for the purpose of genetic testing is not of benefit in itself, since the ethical and social disadvantages could outweigh the advantages. Following this criticism from Denmark and other countries, the EEC programme was modified, and it was decided to include an analysis of its possible ethical consequences.

In autumn 1990, the Danish Council of Ethics issued a report on the ethical aspects of fetal diagnosis, including genetic testing, stating that, in Denmark, fetal diagnosis should have the sole purpose of detecting severe diseases. The Council did not specify what illnesses should be considered severe, since it thought it impossible to draw up a list of genetic and other illnesses or defects which would make abortion ethically defensible and which would not. The Council regarded the use of fetal diagnosis as unacceptable if it was done to pursue eugenic or economic objectives, or to establish the sex or the presence of normal genetic traits in the fetus in order to choose the same by elimination through abortion. The 17-member council could not agree on all of the ethical questions involved in genetic testing of fetuses. Thirteen members argued that the woman has the right to be given all available genetic information about her fetus on request. Four members argued that information regarding normal genetic traits or sex should not be given to the woman until the end of the 12th week of pregnancy, thereby excluding free abortion. The report was submitted to the Danish Minister of Health, the parliamentary Committee on the Council of Ethics, the Health Committee of Parliament, and other MPs. It was not discussed widely in Parliament, but a number of MPs, especially from the Christian Party, took part in a public debate by writing or giving interviews in the press. The report has not resulted in a new regulation issued by the Ministry of Health, but new guidelines are expected.

In 1990, the National Board of Health under the Minister of Health released a report on screening, including genetic screening. It was written by a nonpolitical expert group, and recommended that the WHO guidelines on screening should be followed. It also suggested that the ethical and psychological consequences, including stigmatization, should be evaluated before a screening programme was started, and argued that an economic evaluation should take place. The report was not discussed by the Parliament, but was taken into consideration by the Council of Ethics in its report on genetic screening in 1993.

In 1992, the Council of Ethics published its report "Protection of sensitive information about persons, especially genetic information". In this report, the Council said that the integrity of man should always be protected. The Council concluded that sensitive information about a person should be registered only with the informed consent of the person concerned, unless specific legislation allows otherwise. Together with the Committee on the Council of Ethics, the Council arranged a conference on the premises of Parliament to discuss the report with researchers, organizations and administrative bodies.

In 1993, the Council of Ethics issued a report on "Genetic Screening", which recommended that all genetic screening projects should be ethically evaluated by the Central Scientific Committee as well as by the Council of Ethics itself. (The Central Scientific Committee heads seven regional committees, which must approve all medical research involving human beings.) The

Council also formulated principles for the information of persons to be tested, and for the evaluation of the consequences of genetic screening.

The Danish Board of Technology

The Danish Board of Technology was established in 1986. Its members are appointed by Parliament, and the Board is thus independent of the Government and the Civil Service. According to the law on the Board of Technology, the board has the purposes 1) of following and initiating technology assessment in order to analyse the consequences of new technology for the society and the members of the society, and 2) of creating public debate on these issues. The Board of Technology should try to establish a future-orientated basis for debates on technological issues in Parliament and among the general public. The Board should set out the possibilities of future developments, and bring arguments to the debate, but should not propose legal regulations. Thus the Board was to be independent of special interests, and was to work closely together with Parliament, and the latter could use the results of its work.

The Board has its parliamentary connection through a 9 members committee of MPs which has the task of appointing the 15 Board members. The parliamentary Committee is also involved in the formulation of the broader issues to be analysed by the Board of Technology, and helps to plan the work programme some years ahead. Thus, some of the activities of the Board of Technology arise from a consultation with the parliamentary Committee, or sometimes with the parliamentary Committee on Science and Technology. Of the 15 members of the Board of Technology, the chairperson and 3 members are appointed directly by the parliamentary Committee and 11 are nominated by the following interest groups: 3 by the National Research Councils, 2 by the Association for the Education of the Danish people, and one each by other organizations such as the trade unions, the employers' association, municipal organizations, and the consumers' organization. The Board of

Technology is charged with making reports and technology assessments in fields such as ecology, traffic, environmental issues, health technology and information technology.

Consensus Conferences

One way to explore different aspects of new technology is to arrange consensus conferences. In these, it is lay people and not experts who evaluate new technologies, after they have questioned experts in a certain field. The 15 lay people are volunteers selected to represent the adult Danish population. The lay panel formulates questions, which are presented to the experts in advance. After a two day questioning of experts, the lay people are alone for the weekend to make their report. The panel has to try to establish a consensus. The report is then read aloud to the experts, the audience and the press. The experts can correct misunderstandings, but cannot influence the views expressed in the report.

The Board of Technology also publishes debate-books, movies, video cassettes and magazines in order to generate public debate on issues of technology asssessment. It also subsidizes local public meetings on the assessment of technology. In the years 1987-90 a biotechnological research and development programme was established in Denmark: 21 m DKR were spent on information and technology assessment. Among the issues analysed were mapping of the human genome, ethics and biotechnology etc. These activities were administered by the Board of Technology.

The Board of Technology informs the Parliament about its work and about new technical developments of political interest. Thus, following the Board of Technology's consensus conferences, the final document with recommendations from the conference laymens' panel is sent to all MPs. So are other reports, books and brochures resulting from the the work of the Board. MPs are also informed by news letters from the Board of Technology to the Danish Parliament about technology assessment issues in general, as well as about specific projects of technology assessment initiated by the Board itself. The Danish Board of Technology has released several publications on biotechnology, such as mapping of the human genome, and, in 1989, it arranged a consensus conference on the human genome project. The Board has carried out an analysis of public attitudes towards biotechnology, and an analysis of the public debate. In 1992, it published a report on biotechnology and public debate in the USA, Germany and Britain.

EPTA

The Danish Board of Technology is participating in the European Parliamentary Technology Assessment network (EPTA) along with five other European technology assessment offices with a close relation to parliaments: the German TAB, the Dutch NOTA, the French OPECST, the British POST, and the European Parliament's STOA. EPTA has arranged a conference on bioethics at which the Danish Board of Technology presented its consensus conference concept, and the results of its consensus conference on mapping of the human genome. It was decided to work further on bioethical questions such as the registration of information on human genetic traits, and gene therapy.

Parliamentary information about HIV/AIDS testing

Although the Danish Parliament has established independent bodies to inquire about bioethical issues and technology assessment, the way it is informed about the social and ethical issues in HIV/AIDS testing follows more traditional bureaucratic lines. In 1986, the National Board of Health, which is a branch of the Ministry of Health, established an AIDS secretariat to head the national effort to prevent the spread of AIDS by informing the general public, and risk groups, about preventive measures. The AIDS secretariat has initiated several information campaigns, and also supports local AIDS committees and interest groups in their efforts to spread information. Information from the Secretariat on ethical and social issues in AIDS prevention is reported to the Minister of Health and the Health Committee in Parliament, which is the permanent parliamentary committee dealing with this issue. The AIDS Secretariat publishes a news magazine on AIDS, several times a year, which is sent to all the members of Parliament. The MPs also receive yearly reports from the AIDS Secretariat on the HIV position in Denmark and on preventive strategies.

An important source of information to Parliament is the National Danish Organization for Gays and Lesbians. The Organization publishes a magazine and a newsletter, which are sent to the Health Committee, the Legislative Committee and the Labour Market Committee in Parliament. Yearly reports and reports on specific issues are also sent to the Parliament.

The general principles of the Danish HIV/AIDS preventive strategy were set out by Parliament following a major debate in 1987. The debate followed several questions to the Minister of Interior in the year 86/87 from MPs wanting a register of HIV-positive people and AIDS patients. In a question to the Minister of Interior, the opposition asked what measures the government would take in the fight against AIDS. Following the debate, a majority representing a broad spectrum of the political parties, with only 2 votes against, decided on the following principles: Danish efforts against AIDS should be based on the voluntary principle, anonymity, open and direct information, individual confidentiality in contacting the health authorities, and the avoidance of discrimination. Along these lines, Parliament wanted more resources directed to information for young people, and more support to preventive measures in especially vulnerable groups.

In the following years, some MPs, especially from one right wing party, raised questions in Parliament challenging the 1987 principles. They concerned health workers' contact with HIV-positive persons, and the possibility of registering HIV-positive individuals. In 1991 a right wing party proposed a law on the registration of HIV-positive individuals and AIDS patients. According to this party, the purpose was to improve surveillance of the spread of HIV infection. It was also argued that HIV infected persons in the register could be contacted immediately if there were new treatment possibilities. Only one of the parties in Parliament voted for this proposal.

Thus in Denmark, HIV testing only takes place with the informed consent of the tested person, and a person can be tested without revealing his name. The only group screened for HIV antibodies at the moment is blood donors; this group has been screened since 1986. All cases of AIDS are registered by name, and all HIV-positive cases are reported anonymously by the doctors to the State Serum Institute with information on sex, age, county of residence, and possible way of infection. The only purpose of this registration is epidemiological.

In the last few years, the principles of the Danish HIV preventive strategies have not been changed. In 1992, however, the Chief Medical Officer argued in a particular case for disclosure of information about a person's HIV-positive status in the interest of others, and some MPs took part in the public debate. As a result of the debate, the National Board of Health specified that information on HIV-positive patients cannot be disclosed except in the interest of another person, *e.g.* if there is an obvious risk of transmission of HIV infection to a partner and the HIV-positive person does not want to inform the partner. Information cannot be disclosed to another health care person, as there is no obvious risk of transmission if general preventive measures are followed.

Legal measures

Legal measures regulating genetic testing and screening

Prenatal genetic testing is regulated not by law but by a guidance of April 21st 1981 from the Danish National Board of Health, containing rules on the methods of sampling, indications, and genetic counselling. Women at risk of bearing children with chromosomal diseases, congenital metabolic diseases or other congenital malformations are offered fetal diagnosis. Serious diseases and genetic disorders are listed as examples of those to be tested for. Certain risk groups are defined which should be offered prenatal testing, *e.g.* women who have already borne children with genetic diseases or severe handicaps, and women over 35 years of age.

Following discussions in Parliament in the early eighties on the possibilities of misuse of medical science, Law no. 353 of July 3rd 1987 establishing the Danish Council of Ethics prohibited certain genetic experiments such as those aimed at creating genetically identical human beings, or human beings made by fusing genetically different fetuses, or human beings with a mixture of genetic material from different species. These prohibitions have now been transferred to Law no. 503 of July 24th 1992 concerning a system of research ethics committees and the hearing of biomedical research projects. At the moment, nothing prohibits an insurance company from asking applicants for results from an earlier genetic test, or from asking the applicant to be genetically tested before insurance is granted.

Danish law regulating the labour market gives the employer the right to know an applicant's health condition, and this might include the test results from genetic testing. No law prohibits a private employer from asking an applicant to be genetically tested before employment.

The fact that the use of genetic testing in insurance and in the labour market is not regulated caused the Minister of Labour in 1991 to introduce a bill prohibiting any use of genetic testing in insurance or in the labour market. The bill gave rise to several debates in Parliament, it was criticized by some for being too strict because employees could benefit from genetic testing, if their work environment or work conditions were to change as a result. The bill only regulated DNA testing, and some MPs stated that susceptibility could be tested by other means as well. It was reintroduced by the Minister of Labour in 1992, and another bill on the same issue was proposed in 1993 by a left wing party. After a public hearing in 1993 a committee was set up by the Minister of Labour. The committee has to make proposals for legislation on genetic testing for appointments and for the writing pensions and insurance. Among others, the Danish Council of Ethics is represented on the committee.

Legal regulation relevant to HIV testing

Under order no. 1012 of December 14th 1993 from the National Board of Health, all cases of AIDS are registered by name at the State Serum institute, as are other cases of serious infectious diseases, and all HIV-positive cases must be reported anonymously by doctors to that institute, with information on sex, age, county of residence, and possible means of infection. HIV testing can take place anonymously, and, according to Danish law, civil servants are bound by professional secrecy concerning this information.

All patients must give their informed consent before an HIV test is done, under an order dated September 22nd 1992 from the National Board of Health.

The only HIV-screening taking place in Denmark at the moment is screening of blood donors, which was started in 1986 and is now done under a circular from the National Board of Health dated June 1st 1988.

Conclusion

The Danish parliament has a well established information system in the field of genetic testing and screening, and in other bioethical issues. MPs can ask questions of the Minister of Health or other relevant ministers, who are obliged to answer within days. Special permanent committees of parliament, the Health Committee and the committees on the ethical Council and the Board of Technology, continuously receive information from the Council of Ethics and the Board of Technology, and can ask the Council and the Board to analyse issues of interest to Parliament. In the field of HIV/AIDS, the Parliament is informed by the national Board of Health. Members of Parliament will also be informed by their personal political networks and by the press.

Appendix

The Danish Parliament (Folketinget) has one House. At the moment, the 179 members represent eight parties. The parties are represented proportional to the share of the votes at the elections.

Bioethics in the French Parliament

BERNARD RULLIER [1]

It is worth noting that, in France as in the other great European democracies, modern parliamentary rules give the government very important handles to intervene in the parliament. Thus under the Constitution of 4 October 1958, and in contradiction with the Republican tradition which prevailed under preceding regimes, the Government lays down the parliamentary agenda and can control the Parliament's right of amendment. Moreover, although the right to initiate legislation is accorded under the Constitution to every member of Parliament, law is, in practice, essentially of governmental origin, and is thus administrative.

In France, parliamentary interest in bioethics has met two obstacles. First, the very principle of legislative intervention has long been contested and still is. Secondly, the creation of a National Consultative Ethics Committee by presidential decree in 1983 has allowed Parliament, as it were, to get out of its responsibility in this matter, although the Committee, enjoying moral authority only, and having no more than consultative power, may do no more than give opinions.

---

1. Administrator in the French Senate.

General

The institutions which can be referred to about the ethical questions arising from screening for HIV and genetic disease in the French Senate and National Assembly are as follows:

— Permanent Committees of the two Houses, which can hear a case put by a minister (for example the Minister of Health) or a senior civil servant (for example the Permanent Secretary at the Ministry of Health); or examine the text of a bill, for instance one to regulate the use of genetic tests or to forbid discrimination based on the presence of genetic or other diseases.

— Research and documentation services:

• The Information Service of the Senate and the Documentation Service of the National Assembly answer inquiries from parliamentarians, provided they are precise and relevant.

• The Comparative Legislation Service of the Senate carries out general studies on the legislation of the principal member states of the EC, and of the Western world.

• The Parliamentary Office for the Evaluation of Scientific Choices (OPECST).

Nevertheless, the French Parliament has no specific organ which would enable it to tackle bioethical questions over time and in a multidisciplinary way.

Internal

Preparatory documentation to parliamentary discussion

In December 1986, the French government commissioned the Council of State to make a study called "From Ethics to Law". It was received in February 1988 and published immediately. In September 1988, the new government set up an interdisciplinary interministerial working group charged with putting the Council of State's proposals into legislative form (except those concerning experimentation on people, since those were already dealt with in bills then going through parliament). This working group then prepared a draft bill on life sciences and human rights, which was submitted to the Prime Minister in April 1989. Though it was not published, it was fairly widely distributed in parliamentary circles.

But this text was given up; it was neither laid before the Council of State nor adopted by the Council of Ministers, both of which are necessary if a text is to become a bill and to be placed before the two Houses of Parliament.

The preliminary debate on bioethical legislation was started again in 1990 by two initiatives. The first, from the Socialist Senator Franck Serusclat, led to the Parliamentary Office for the Evaluation of Scientific and Technological Choices becoming refered to about the matter. The second was the setting up of an Information Mission on Bioethics in the National Assembly *(see below)*.

At the same time, in October 1990 the government charged Mme Noelle Lenoir, a senior civil servant, with the task of producing the new report. This report, which was entitled "At the Frontiers of Life: for a New Biomedical Ethic *à la Francaise*" was supported by 24 contributions from scientific experts, by public hearings of "eminent witnesses" (research scientists, parliamentarians, representatives of the churches) and by a synopsis of comparative law.

On the basis of the parliamentary work thus far, and of the Lenoir report, three bills were drafted by the civil service (the Health Department at the Ministry of Social Affairs, and the Chancellery at the Ministry of Justice) and were adopted by the Council of Ministers on 25 March 1992.

— Bill N° 2599:
• provided a legal framework for the protection of the human

body and wrote it into the Civil Code,
* regulated the use of genetic tests,
* established, through clear rules, the validity of paternity in the case of medically-assisted pregnancy.

— Bill N° 2600:
* wrote general principles governing the giving and using of elements and products of the human body into the Civil Code,
* reformed the Loi Caillavet of 1976 on the removal of organs,
* brought medically-assisted procreation and prenatal diagnoses within the Code of Public Health,
* introduced considerable administrative and penal sanctions.

— Bill N° 2601:
* introduced a specific regime for research data in Public Health, superseding Law No. 78-17 of 6 January 1978 on information, records and freedoms.

The members of Parliament who were working on biomedical ethics were not formally associated or consulted on the editing of these texts that were, however, laid before them in an outline at an informal meeting on 17 December 1991, and were the subject of a government communication of 18 December 1991.

Besides government reports, documentation preliminary to parliamentary discussion takes two forms in France. The first is the documentation prepared for the legislative debate itself. Every White Paper or bill is sent to a permanent committee, which designates a rapporteur. While the text of the 1958 Constitution intended that texts should be sent before special ad hoc committees, parliamentary practice has actually been the contrary: there have been permanent committees, whose number is limited to six by the Constitution, which study all the White Papers and bills that are sent to them. Thus the setting up of a special committee in the National Assembly to study the three bills *(see above)* was a rather exceptional procedure, to which attention should be drawn.

A rapporter, helped by one or more members of the parliamentary staff, holds hearings and produces a public report in which he examines the general thrust of the text, and proposes, if he thinks fit, its modification by amendments which will thereafter be discussed in the committee and then at a public session.

The French parliament is also endowed with particular organs of information, preliminary to, or independent of all legislative debate.

They consist principally of:

— the parliamentary office, OPECST *(see below)*,
— the delegation of the National Assembly to the European Communities that has, for example, published an information paper on the Commission Directive of 14 June 1989 concerning medical products derived from human blood plasma,
— the Comparative Law Unit of the European Secretariat of the Senate, which has published studies on euthanasia, the right to abortion, medically-assisted procreation (January 1991) and regulations concerning the use of embryos (April 1991).

The activities of the permanent committees of the Assemblies

The three above mentioned bills were examined in the National Assembly by a special committee set up on 22 April 1992.

The committee met in May and June 1992 (twelve meetings including ministerial hearings). It proceeded to a detailed examination of the three bills, and adopted them after substantial modifications in a report published on 30 March 1992.

The National Assembly examined these texts in public session during five days: 19, 20, 23, 24 and 25 November 1992.

The texts were transmitted to the Senate on 26 November 1992.

They are still under examination, because the progress of bills on bioethics, which had passed their first reading in the National Assembly, has been suspended because of the paliamentary election of March 1993. They were not put on the order paper for the spring session: the government judged that they were not of sufficient legislative urgency. Besides, the government seems to be doubtful about the method followed up till then, namely the splitting up of bioethical questions into three separate texts.

Work in committee has been undertaken in the Senate during the spring term of 1993, but in an uncertain rhythm. It has been going ahead in the Committee on Social Affairs, but has remained modest in the Legal Committee. The committee meetings examining these texts have not been open to the public. A summary record of the discussions and the hearings of committees is nonetheless published in the Committee Bulletin which is received by every Member of Parliament, and can be diffused outside.

The work of the Senate Committees of 1993 on bioethical texts has been as follows:

— The Legal Committee has appointed Mr. M. Cabanel (human body) and Mr. Turk (epidemiological records) as the rapporteurs on the bill. On 5 May 1993, it heard Mr. Glorion, the new chairman of the Council of the Order (of physicians), Mr. Changeux, the new chairman of the National Consultative Committee on Ethics, Mr. Jean Bernard, and Mr. Schiele, a Senator and a member of the National Committee on "Information and Freedom".

— The Social Affairs Committee has held about 30 hearings since the beginning of spring 1993.

— The Cultural Affairs Committee appointed Mr. P.L. Lafitte on 7 April 1993 as the rapporteur on the bill concerning the donation of gametes, prenatal diagnostics, medically-assisted procreation and on the National Consultative Committee on Ethics.

Committees of inquiry

Two committees of inquiry have dealt in the French Parliament with questions on biomedical ethics.

— **The Bioulac report on behalf of the special committee of the National Assembly concerning bioethics:**

An information mission on bioethics was set up in October 1990 by the National Assembly. It was composed of members of the Committee on Cultural, Family and Social Affairs and the Legal Committee and was chaired by Bernard Bioulac, a socialist deputy for Dordogne and a neuro-physiologist.

It held about 15 hearings between December 1990 and April 1991, at which were heard about 60 people, then seven gathered round table discussions which were open to persons not belonging to the Mission: the debates were published in the Rapport de l'Information between May and July 1991.

The congestion of the autumn session delayed the publication of the report till 18 February 1992.

Those debates showed that the search for consensus on these questions was difficult. Which questions should or should not be the subject of legislation (which was the question that led to the creation of this Information Mission) as well as the content of any legislation there might be, were bitterly discussed among the members of the Commission.

— **The committees of inquiry on the transfusion system ("the contaminated blood scandal"):**

A committee of inquiry of the Senate on the system of transfusion was set up on 17 December 1991 and reported on 12 June 1992. It grappled with the ethical aspects of the drama of the contamination of transfusion blood by the AIDS virus. About 30 public hearings were held.

During the winter of 1992/93, the National Assembly adopted the same procedure and set up its own committee of inquiry concentrating on scientific knowledge about AIDS.

Informal committees

In both Houses there are study groups, as for example the study group on "Life Sciences" in the Senate, or that on "Questions Airising from the Advance of Medicine", which could tackle biomedical ethics. They organize hearings and working lunches but are only moderately active.

Initiatives by individual members of Parliament

As noted above, laws which start in Parliament have been rare in France since 1958: they represent only about 10% of the texts. It is thus exceptional that the major laws about biomedical ethics should be of parliamentary origin, like the law of 22 December 1976 concerning removal of organs which was proposed by Senator Henri Caillavet, or the law of 20 December 1988 proposed by Senator Claude Huriet and taken up by Senator Franck Serusclat.

The French Parliament has, in fact, never neglected the juridical questions posed by the progress of medicine and biology.

The case of medically assisted procreation is particularly instructive. When the law of 3 January 1972 on paternity was discussed in Parliament, the question of artificial insemination was raised in the National Assembly during the discussion of Articles 340 and 341: these concern investigations into paternity, and are consequently at the heart of discussions on the juridical consequences of medically assisted procreation using donor sperm. One Deputy, Mr. Tissant, pertinently remarked: "The bill was passed over the problem of artificial insemination in silence which, at least in the case of an insemination by a man other than the husband, could be likened to intercourse with another man. The question would be difficult to settle, unless indeed the code of medical ethics were to regulate it." This observation, which alas remained without consequence, is perhaps remarkable, considering that the CECOS[2] were not set up until two years later and that artificial insemination (donor) in

---

2. Centres for the Study and Conservation of Ova and Sperm, which were the founders of the practice of artificial insemination (donor).

France was still largely confidential at the beginning of the 70s. It was not until 1980 that the Parliament, actually the Senate, discussed it in public session for the first time.

Senators Caillavet and Mezard tabled their bill on 26 October 1978. It was directly motivated by the birth of Louise Brown in Great Britain the year before, the first successful *in vitro* fertilization. The importance of this bill lies in the process by which it was drafted. Its authors brought a committee together, called the Society of the Freedoms, under the guidance of the founder of the CECOS, Professor Georges David, which included doctors, psychiatrists and theologians, among whom Father Legrand, the Vice-Rector of the Catholic Institute.

The bill embodies four principles:

— The consents of the couple and the donor are required. It must be informed by an interview with a psychologist and can be withdrawn at any moment.

— The function and the identity of the donor must remain secret.

— The function can only be carried out under the supervision of a doctor, it must have no eugenic or financial purpose, and the sperm must be a free gift.

— Disavowal may not be entertained in law if it is established that the child has been conceived by means of artificial insemination. This provision refers to a judgement of the TGI (Tribunal) of Nice on 30 June 1976, which is explicitly mentioned in the preamble to the bill and was the first judgement to have approved disavowal by the husband in a couple which had had recourse to artificial insemination (donor).

Before the Council of State Report of 1988, three other proposals concerning artificial procreation were laid before Parliament:

— Proposal n° 255 from Senator Henri Caillavet, 8 April 1982. This would have put all the centres carrying out medically assisted procreation within the responsibility of a multidisciplinary "institute of bioethics and human reproduction", including researchers and doctors, "psycho-social experts", and also representatives of Parliament, family associations, and jurists.

— Proposal n° 258 by Mr. Pierre Bas, 18 May 1984. Of unexampled precision, it was intended to provide a framework for research in order to prevent "researchers doing whatever they wanted". It would also have reserved artificial insemination to married couples. Every local health authority was to be endowed with an Ethics Committee, whose members were to give their opinion on research projects and experimental procreation. Penalties were proposed.

— Proposal n° 257 by Senator Francis Palmero, 24 April 1985, "concerning the juridical consequences of post mortem insemination". It would have amended the Civil Code to allow the establishment of paternity after the death of the husband, provided he had stated before an attorney that this was his wish, by extending the presumption of paternity after death to 480 days, thereby modifying Articles 725 and 795 concerning succession in the Civil Code.

This proposal was precipitated by a judgement of the court at Creteil in 1984, which ordered that sperm which was being held by a CECOS should be returned to the widow of the man who had deposited it there, if so requested by the widow.

After the Council of State report "From Ethics to Law" of 1988, the debate on bioethics was relaunched when a number of bills directly or indirectly affecting medically assisted procreation were laid before Parliament.

— **In the National Assembly:**

• N° 1156 from Mme Christine Boutin on 19 December 1989: "To ensure respect for the integrity of the person".

• N° 1976 from Mr. Jean Francois Mattei and others on 2nd April 1991: "A general bill concerning life sciences and respect for man".

- N° 2047 from Mr. Jacques Toubon on 14 May 1991: "Designed to assign penal sanctions to the infringements of the principle of the non-patrimoniality of the human body".

- N° 2106 from Mr. Jacques Toubon on 12 June 1991: "Designed to determine the ethical principles by which the integrity, the identity and the dignity of the person can be protected".

— In the Senate:

- N° 309 from Mr. Bernard Seillier on 22 May 1990: "On the health of the human person".

These bills state rather general principles, treating the question of medically assisted procreation indirectly, and from a rather repressive point of view, in order to prohibit the gift of ovocytes and prohibit surrogate motherhood (Bill N° 1156 by Mme Boutin) and the gift of embryos and surrogate motherhood (Bill N° 309 by Mr. Seillier). The practice of surrogate motherhood is also prohibited in Mr. Mattei's bill, in the name of the integrity of the human body, and in Bill N° 2106 Mr. Toubon, in the name of the inalienability of the human body. Only Bill N° 1156 by Mme Boutin favoured the removal of anonymity from sperm donors.

The most coherent and best worked out bills were laid by Senator Frank Serusclat for the Socialist Group. Two bills dated 25 February 1988, one concerning "the paternity of children born by medically assisted procreation" (N° 237) and the other "the collection, conservation and utilisation of human gametes" (N° 238), which were taken up by the Socialist Group in the National Assembly (under Bill N° 1204), were rounded off by a third bill of 8 July 1988 concerning medically assisted procreation (N° 327).

Bill N° 238 sets out the principles which should govern medically assisted procreation: (1) It must be done only by medically qualified people; (2) gamete donation must not be commercialized; (3) medically assisted procreation centres must be licensed by the Health Minister; (4) the anonymity of the donor must be preserved.

Bill N° 237 modifies the Civil Code so as to institute a new procedure of declaration of consent before a magistrate in order — according to the purposes of the Bill — "to ensure that the couple are properly informed as to the juridical consequences of their consent, and to guarantee the seriousness and reality of their agreement through a private interview with the judge, and a pause for thought of not less than one week". This formality was justified by a concern to "avoid the development of disagreements harmful to the children born through medically assisted procreation". Under this bill, no paternity was to be established in the case of donors of gametes or embryos, and paternity might neither be disavowed, nor disputed, nor recognized, except in order to establish that the child was not the result of what the judge in 1990 called "a voluntarily indeterminate paternity".

Bill N° 327 modified the Code of Public Health in order to regulate the activities of the IVF centres. Those benefiting by IVF — who had to be a heterosexual couple both of whom were alive — had to affirm their consent according to the provisions of the Civil Code as modified by Bill N° 327. Centres practising IVF were to be subject to ministerial licence, "in order to prevent anarchic development and doubtful practices". The principle of free treatment is reaffirmed. Only a *docteur en médecine* or a medical team under his direction can apply these procreative techniques; doctors enjoy a conscience clause which allows them not to participate. The anonymity of the donor of gametes or an embryo is instituted, except for medical reasons.

Thus one can say that during this period, the Parliament was not completely absent from the debate on bioethics, and especially from the questions posed by medically assisted procreation. The plethora of bills — to say nothing of written questions or of the work of various study groups such as the

"Senate Study Group on the Life Sciences" — and the growing awareness in the public mind, of the drawbacks of an unregulated and unsupervised against its own excesses activity, showed that Parliament is the necessary gateway from ethics to law, even if, in some quarters it has been denied that the law has a right or a legitimacy enabling it to deal with social questions.

In May 1993, the new Government entrusted temporary responsibility for "the juridical aspects of research into, and the health of bioethics" to Mr. Jean Francois Mattei, a deputy and a doctor, who had taken an active part in the work of the Bioulac Committee and the legislative debate in the National Assembly. He was to keep the progress of legislative procedures under review (since proposals on bioethics run into medical hostility from an important section of the present Parliamentary majority), to study the consequences of a report from the *Inspection Générale des Affaires Sociales* on human tissue banks and organ donations, and on the application of the law of 20 December 1988.

Now, after two years' examination in Parliament, but more than ten years in preparatory debate, France has finally endowed itself with a legislation on bioethics by two laws on 29 July 1994. They have been submitted to the Constitutional Council, which, on 27 July 1994 found them constitutional. The Council acted on the application of the members of Parliament and also, which is unusual, of the President of the National Assembly himself. In its decision, the Constitutional Council declared that the principle of "he protection of the dignity of the human person against all forms of subjection and degradation" has now a constitutional status.

The first law, number 94-653, on the respect for the human body, modifies both the Civil and the Penal Codes. Its first section writes the principle of the respect for the human body into the Civil Code by a new article 16, which proclaims that "the law guarantees the primacy of the person, prohibits all derogation of the dignity of the person, and guarantees the respect for the human being from the beginning of life".

These principles should be viewed as a proclamation of the inviolable character of the human body and its integrity, neither of which may be infringed except in the case of therapeutic necessity for that person, who must, as a matter of principle, give advance consent. The infringement of the integrity of the human species is also prohibited, as are eugenic practices aiming to the selection of persons.

The law also asserts that the human body, its elements and its products, cannot be the subject of the law of property. Contracts for procreation or gestation on behalf of other people are null; and no remuneration may be given to those who lend themselves for experimentation or for the removal of tissues or organs. Likewise the human body, its elements and products, and the knowledge of the total or partial structure of a human gene are not patentable.

Finally, anonymity is guaranteed to donors and recipients.

The section 2 of the law regulates genetic fingerprinting, which is limited to medical or research aims. It can be used in paternity cases on the order of a judge, and with the prior consent of the concerned person. This section also provides penalties for all the offences created by the two laws.

The section 3 of the Law declares that no bond of paternity can be established, in the case of medically assisted procreation, between the donor and the child born of the procreation. It sets up a prior consent procedure before a judge or a notary.

Law number 94-654, on the gift and use of elements and products of the human body, for the purposes of therapy, procreation, and prenatal diagnosis, changes the Code of Public Health on several points.

It sets up a national register of refusals to permit the removal of organs from deceased persons. It also sets control over establishments practising organ transplants, or the removal of tissues or cells for the purpose of donation.

Public funds for assisted procreation are limited to married couples or to couples who have been living in concubinage for at least two years and have given prior consent. They are also limited to cases of infertility, the pathological character of which has been medically certified. An embryo must be conceived with a gamete from at least one of the couple. Embryos which are not implanted must be kept during five years. At the end of this period, their fate is to be examined again by the law, but those conceived before this law was passed may be destroyed. Embryos may also be given to another couple, by judicial decision and after the advance consent of the donor couple. Experiments on embryos are in principle forbidden, except in the case of the express consent of the couple, the approval of a committee, and for a medical purpose: experiments must not harm the embryos. Establishments which receive public funds for assisted procreation must inform their clients in detail in the course of the interviews.

Insemination with fresh sperm is forbidden, and so is the birth of more than five children from gametes of the same donor. Only non-profit-making establishments may practice medically assisted procreation.

Finally, the genetic characteristics of a person may not be examined except for the purposes of therapy or scientific research.

A parliamentary technology assessment office

The ethical aspects of screening for genetic diseases were studied in the Serusclat report presented on behalf of the Parliamentray Office for the Evaluation of Scientific and Technological Choices (OPECST): by remits dated 25 April 1990 from Laurent Fabius, the chairman of the National Assembly, and 30 May 1990 from Alain Poher, the chairman of the Senate, OPECST — on 19 December 1990 — designated Senator

Frank Serusclat as the rapporteur of a project which was to gather scientific information in order to inform the Parliament of the state of progress in the "life sciences". The report appeared in the form of an ethical discourse, supported by more than 350 hours of interviews and numerous trips abroad, carried out throughout the year. The introduction specifies the rapporteur's method of work. Two days of public hearings also took place at the Senate, on 5 and 6 December 1991.

The report was adopted by OPECST on 4 February and published on 11 February 1992.

The Office is now referred to as regards organ transplants.

The working method of the office is as follows. Under the Article 6(3) of Resolution N° 58-1100 of 17 November 1958, the Parliamentary Office, which was created in 1983, is charged with "informing the parliament of the consequences of choices of a scientific and technological character, principally in order to clarify its decisions. For this purpose it will collect information, institute programmes of study, and proceed to assessments".

The layout of the resolution of 1958 defining the purpose and the responsibilities of the Office and describing the procedures it may use, calls for comment. The Office undertakes parliamentary studies. It never sub-contracts the whole of a report, but produces it in-house. The rapporteurs are parliamentarians. If they need expert advice, it is always available. A rapporteur can also apply to the members of the Scientific Council of the Office, but this procedure is seldom used. An independent expert's advice supports the report in question, it does not replace it. In consequence, the adopted point of view — which is political — can be distinct from the strictly scientific or technological considerations so as to include reflections of a general economic, social or political nature. A report from the Office is elicited by political opportunity, and has to answer two main questions:

— What technological problem is important enough to demand parliament's attention?

— What answer can be given to it, particularly, but not exclusively, on the legislative level?

The Office has no power of automotion. It must be commissioned to produce a report either by the Bureau of one of the chambers of Parliament, which has itself been reffered to about the matter by the chairman of a political group or by 60 deputies or 40 senators, or by a special or permanent Committee. No organism outside Parliament can commission a report, nor can any single parliamentarian.

In addition to the scrutiny by the Bureau, project proposals encounter a second filter with the "feasibility study" which decides the themes and the fields of investigation to be undertaken, as well as the methods.

Automotion was excluded when the Office was set up in 1983, since some members of Parliament feared an encroachment on the roles of the permanent committees.

The Office is only commissioned to study a question in a temporary manner. The consequence of this is that the Office does not have any competence to examine scientific and technological questions in such and such field, on a continuing basis. At the moment, since the adoption of the Serusclat report, the Office has not been under instruction to study any question of bioethics, and no running commission has been established by the Parliament, despite the fact that the relevant scientific progress is advancing rapidly, particularly in the cartography of the human genome.

The functions of the Office are strictly limited by those of the legislative procedure. In other words, whether in bioethics or in any other subject, it cannot substitute its own work for that of the professional organizations (for instance medical) or of the major advisory commissions (the National Consultative Committee on Ethics, the High Council for Population and the

Family...) and it cannot keep an eye on public research organizations such as INSERM or the National Research Council from the point of view of the ethical implications of their research.

The competence of the Office is implicitly limited to the problems which arise in the legislative domain, and which naturally precede the examination of a bill by the relevant committees of Parliament.

— The composition of the Office:

• The Office is only composed of parliamentarians, who are the rapporteurs for the studies which it carries out.

• The membership of the Office is half and half, as between the two assemblies, and is politically balanced according to the representation of political groups under the proportional electoral law.

• Parliamentary rapporteurs are usually alone in handling a research project, occasionally two; they are assisted by administrators from the staff of the two Chambers. Besides they can have recourse to experts, which is fairly common. The latter are remunerated by the Office, which is financed by the two Chambers.

• It is worthy of note that Senator Serusclat rejected this method, so as not to link his opinion to that of a scientific expert, who might thus have appeared as a spokesman for one of the factions in the debate, one of the stakes being precisely the freedom of research.

— The methods of work of the Office: They are governed by internal minutes of 20 November and December 1984, as follows: "After the Office has been commissioned to undertake a project, and a rapporteur has been appointed, there shall first be carried out a feasibility study and report, which could conclude that it would be inopportune to pursue the study": that happened with AIDS. After that, a study of methodology and a work programme are drawn up, only after which, and on the basis of which, the study itself can begin in the form of collective expertise grouped around the parliamentary rapporteur and gathering specialists in different fields, an ad hoc working group if the rapporteur so wishes, and of course the multidisciplinary Council of the Office draws up an opinion on the draft of the final report. Once they are approved, the reports are in principle published and are wound up with recommendations constituting the decisive element, or, at any rate, a significant element of the work which has been done.

Existence of a specialized library

The parliament does not have a library specializing in the questions of biomedical ethics.

Periodicals carried in the libraries

The libraries of the two chambers subscribe to general scientific periodicals and to popular science periodicals such as *La Recherche, Science et Vie*, and *Science et Avenir*. The Senate library has just acquired a "Permanent Dictionary of Bioethics and Biotechnologies".

The Parliamentary Office receives the English language periodicals *Science* and *Nature*. It disposes of a rather limited documentation fund, since the documentation is acquired as and when, according to the studies which are required.

Access to general (press) information and to juridical documentation (laws and regulations, jurisprudence) is a great deal easier than access to scientific or technological information, which is still difficult.

In fact, as to studies in bioethics, the documentation base is practically non-existent, whether in the the Office or the library of the two Chambers.

Access to data banks

The Parliament is connected with *Medline* and Bioethic, but they are never consulted.

Existence of specialized personnel

There is no specialized personnel having a scientific or medical formation in the two chambers of the parliament, and persons having such a formation are not necessarily brought to bear on the inquiries or legislative texts dealing with these questions.

Recourse to outside advisers

The utilisation of experts is practised only in the Parliamentary Office. They can nevertheless be called to hearings according to their qualities.

External

Informing the general public

In addition to the written parliamentary reports, the effort of the two houses at communication has led them to attempt a new stage of transparency: to open the work of the committees to the public, and to organize public hearings. The publication of important reports is now also accompanied by press conferences.

Colloquia can also be organized on the premises of parliament, like the colloquium at the Senate on 13 April 1993 on "Organ Transplants: from ethics to law", organized by Senator Huriet.

To widen the diffusion of its work and its reports, the office has organized numerous public hearings such as those dedicated to biomedical ethics on 5 and 6 December 1991, and has tried to boost the diffusion of parliamentary reports among the general public by printing them in a less austere form, through the publishers "Economica", who specialize in university books.

But the instruction of the general public is given by the National Consultative Committee on Ethics by means of:

— a periodical of information,
— "annual ethics days" open to the public, and decentralized throughout the country,
— the annual publication by the French Government Publishing Office of the collection of opinions given by the Committee.

Activity of outside organisms

In addition to the Ethics Committee mentioned above, the other institution which formally deals with questions of biomedical ethics is the National Council of the medical profession, which has taken up positions on medically assisted procreation and on prenatal diagnostics. The Council of the Profession *(Conseil de l'Ordre)* also organized a very important conference on biomedical ethics on 9 and 10 March 1991, which gathered more than 2,000 doctors and researchers at the Palais des Congrès. The proceedings of the conference were widely diffused.

Links between Parliament and the churches

Because of the formal separation of the churches from the state, which has constitutional status through the law of 1905, there is no official organic relationship between parliament and any of the churches. On the other hand, nothing prevents the churches from asking to be heard at public hearings, and they often do.

Links with academies and universities

These are not institutionally organized, except for the presence of two parliamentarians on the National Consultative Ethics Committee.

Pressure groups

Pressure groups are not recognized as such by the French Parliament, because of the representative nature of the parliamentary mandate which prohibits any specific mandate. This principle does not keep them from being heard within the framework of the Office, or at public hearings before the Committees.

Among the most active pressure groups are scientific circles, notably in research, the Catholic Church, and the National Union of Family Associations. The latter have found powerful allies in the new parliamentary majority in their opposition to the legalization of medically assisted procreation and prenatal diagnoses.

Content

The ethical message conveyed by all these reports, proposals, and successive versions of bills, is essentially unitary. It is founded on Roman Law, and the philosophy of the Rights of Man.

From the former, it takes the fundamental distinction, the *summa divisio*, between persons and things. Persons, and also their organs, their products, and their extensions before birth and after death, cannot become the objects of private property, of purchase or sale. Nobody, in principle, may dispose of them, except as expressly provided by the law.

The principles of the inviolability of the human person, the right to a private life, to health, and to information flow from the philosophical corpus of the Enlightenment. The two principle corollaries are consent, and free gift. Several principles derive from that:

— any legitimate invasion of a person requires his or her consent,

— the body itself and all its components cannot be goods,

— experiments on, removals from, and interventions in the human body may have only scientific or therapeutic aims, and not industrial or commercial aims.

These particularly important general rules are held to have been written into the Civil Code, which is the foundation of French private law, and this shows the importance of the implications of biomedial ethics for law.

In the absence, before 1994, of a law or laws in controversial fields like medically assisted procreation, prenatal diagnoses, the removal of organs, and epidemiological records, several minor provisions, of limited application, and sometimes voted in a hurry, there can be listed:

— the Law of 20 December 1988 on the protection of the persons willing to be the subjects of biomedical research. It derives from the bill of Senators Claude Huriet and Franck Serusclat;

— the Law of 12 July 1990 intended to write into the penal Code, the Labour Code, and the 1983 Statute on Public Functions, measures of protection for persons who might suffer from discrimination on grounds of health or handicap. The surrounding discussion was largely about AIDS;

— article 13 of the Law on 31 December 1991, which was extremely controversial, was part of a bill including various social measures. It prohibited insemination with fresh sperm, guaranteed that sperm should be a free gift, and regulated the administrative control of medically assisted procreation by going back to a "tabula rasa" through the withdrawal of existing authorisations, and their replacement by new ones. This provision was much criticized as a hole-and-corner way of legalizing a system of administrative control of medically assisted procreation which wrongly anticipated the legislative proposals of Lenoir Report;

— article 18 of Law N° 31-1477 ON 31 December 1992 on products subject to controls on their sale, and on the uniformity of treatment of such products by the Police, the Gendarmerie and the Customs, subjected "organs, tissues, and gametes taken from the human body" to control by the Minister of Health;

— in the Law of 3 January 1993 amending the Civil Code on marital status, family, and the rights of children, and setting up Family Courts, the Senate deleted a section which prohibited any enquiry into paternity in the case of medically asssisted procreation by a third-party donor, holding that such things should find a place in the bill on the human body;

— the Law of 4 January 1993, on the safety of blood transfusions and of medication, gave an opportunity to reaffirm the principles of benevolence, voluntariness, anonymity, and the absence of profit, already present in the Public Health Code. Following the contaminated blood scandal, the bill made profound changes in the French blood transfusion system, particularly by setting up a "French Blood Agency" and a committee for transfusion safety, thus re-establishing the protection of the state.

Structure and processes of information acquisition in the German Parliament : AIDS and "Genetic Engineering/ Genetic Testing"[1]

THOMAS PETERMANN[2], EDGAR GÖLL[2]

Overview of the working and consultative (advisory) structures at the German Bundestag

This section outlines the consultative and advisory structures at the German Parliament ("Deutscher Bundestag"), broken down according to the various levels and working units. The chief sources of information and briefing available to these are described.

---

1. This report should be considered as a rather statistical, quantitative and descriptive presentation of the structure and processes of information acquisition at the German Parliament (Bundestag). We must point out that two things have not been attempted:
— The present status report does not make any evaluation of the situation or provide any evaluative conclusions. Similarly, the identified information and advisory processes are not reviewed as to their contents and their impacts.
— The reconstruction and description of the two case studies refer to the policy issues AIDS and Genetic Engineering/Genetic Testing in general. It was not possible to isolate the sub-aspects of testing and screening.
2. German Parliament Bureau for the Evaluation of the Consequences of Technology (TAB).

The Plenary Assembly

1. The functions and tasks of the Plenary Assembly of the Bundestag. The Plenary Assembly is the assembly of members, and is the central organ of the federal corporate body called the Deutsche Bundestag. In the final instance, it possesses all decision-making competences. The function of the debates held there (which in principle are always open to the public) is the public exchange of opinions and arguments between the members of parliament and the parliamentary political groups and groupings. The plenary debates are, therefore, the expression and vehicle of communicative democracy.

2. The instruments of the Plenary Assembly

— The parliamentary interpellation: There are different ways of organizing communication and information acquisition in the plenary. Special mention should be made of the major interpellation *(Große Anfrage)* and the minor interpellation *(Kleine Anfrage)*. Both can be submitted by a parliamentary party or at least 5 % of the members of the Bundestag. To a major interpellation a written response has to be given by the government, and it is then debated in the plenary. There are no set time limits. Parliamentary interpellations usually cover issues of general political significance. They refer to the area of responsibility of the government.

A minor interpellation only requires a written reply by the Federal Government within 14 days, and must not automatically be debated. Such interpellations generally cover very specific subjects.

Parliamentary political groups (Fraktionen)

1. Functions and tasks: The parliamentary political groups are a direct expression of the quantitative strength of a party in the Bundestag as established by elections to the Bundestag. In parliament, they are the extended arm of the parties. Consequently, they are interested in projecting their image, in applying their party political programmes in parliament and, not least, in improving their chances for future election success. The parliamentary political groups formulate their political will, which is usually commonly shared by members of the group. The functions of these groups can be summarized as: cooperating with their parties, coordinating parliamentary party group work and government policy (in the governing group), cooperating with the Land governments headed by their parties (parties in opposition) and maintaining contacts with the media, associations and interest groups.

In regard to power and influence, the parliamentary political groups are the chief sub-division of the Bundestag. Only they possess the major parliamentary powers. The parliamentary groups discuss, prestructure and decide on all major issues and strategies of the members of parliament and the committees (*e.g.* legislative proposals/bills, major interpellations, apply-ing for hearings).

The Bureau of the German Bundestag *(Ältestenrat)* decides on the appointments to the committees, the agenda for the plenary sessions, the speaking times etc. The Bureau consists of the President of the Bundestag, the Parliamentary Secretaries and members of the parliamentary groups.

To process work on individual policy issues, the parliamentary groups set up working groups or working parties *(Arbeitsgruppen, Arbeitskreise)* which largely reflect the division of labour in the Bundestag Committees or Federal Ministries. The Working Group members generally belong to the corresponding specialized committee.

2. The instruments of the parliamentary groups

— The parliamentary group services: To assist them in their work, the Bundestag parliamentary groups have set up their own parliamentary group support services, separate from those of the Bundestag administration. In addition to providing administrative and technical support, these parliamentary group support services are structured in staffers of the parliamentary group working parties and working groups, personal assistants to the leadership of the parliamentary group and the parliamentary group's own press office and information services. Their function is to acquire information and make this information available to their group and its members. The parliamentary group's staff are of particular importance for parliamentary groups who are in the opposition (parties), because, in contrast to the groups in the government coalition (parties), these cannot expect great support for their information demands from the ministerial bureaucracy.

The parliamentary group support services provide information to the different working parties and working groups of the parliamentary groups and their executive committees. At the end of 1991 (12th legislative term) the parliamentary groups employed 247 reference and research staff members and 480 other staff members and

— CDU/CSU: 85 reference and research and 195 general staff,
— SPD: 100 reference and research and 190 general staff,
— FDP: 29 reference and research and 58 general staff,
— Group PDS/Left List: 16 reference and research and 26 general staff,
— Alliance 90/The Greens: 17 reference and research and 11 general staff.

— Studies and comments: To support them in their work, the parliamentary group support services and the parliamentary groups occasionally commission expert opinions and comments from external scientists and experts.

Permanent committees (Fachausschüsse)

1. Functions and tasks: At the beginning of each legislative term the Bundestag establishes so-called preparatory decision-making organs, particularly the permanent committees, for the duration of the entire legislative term. These specialized committees are structured to reflect the organization of the Federal Government; each federal ministry is generally confronted with a specialized committee.

The 24 permanent committees of the Bundestag at present fulfil two main functions. They work out bills and other drafts *(Beschlußvorlagen)* and present them to the plenary session of the Bundestag for its decision-making. They also deal with other issues arising in their area. Their function, therefore, is to oversee the activities of the government and/or of the individual ministries.

The bulk of the work of the legislature is carried out in the committees, where the working parties in the parliamentary groups will already have prepared drafts, and will have worked out the general line of political argument. Committee meetings are usually not open to the public.

The members of parliament are appointed members of the committees by the parliamentary groups in relation to the number of MPs they have. Each committee has a secretariat responsible almost exclusively for organization and administrative tasks. It usually consists of one or two members of the higher civil service, a clerk and two typists. The committees do not have a reference or research staff.

2. The instruments of the committees

— Comments and studies: Written or verbal comments and information provided by external scientists and experts (Federal Government and Ministries, Bundesrat and Land Governments, foundations, associations, universities, institutes) are the basic means of information used by the committees. External expertise and representatives of associations can be called in to the working sessions.

— Hearings: In order to obtain information on major consultative issues with large potential for conflict, generally in connection with bills, the committees can invite external experts, representatives of interest groups and other informants

(*Auskunftspersonen*) to public or private hearings. Mostly it is the parliamentary opposition groups who apply for hearings. There is a general trend for hearings to be held in public: (at present three quarters are public). The chairmanship, allotment of time, order of questions and number of experts invited are regulated according to the relative strength of the political parties.

While the hearings serve to obtain information on major specific issues in the legislative process and to integrate scientific expertise and the interest groups involved, they also have the important function of preparing subject-related and political compromises, creating acceptancy and legitimation for majority decisions, improving control possibilities, and the allowing public self projection of the participants. Providing information to the general public is probably of only minor importance.

— Technology Assessment Unit (TAB): The activities of the Technology Assessment Unit of the German Bundestag is based on a resolution of the Bundestag in 1989. TAB receives its commissions primarily from the Committee for Research, Technology and Technology Assessment of the Bundestag, though other committees can also apply. TAB is a special organizational unit of the Karlsruhe Nuclear Research Centre.

Being a scientific unit, TAB's technology-related consultative processes (technology assessment, monitoring of new TA-developments, methods) contribute to improving the Bundestag's information and decision-making. This is achieved by intensive interaction between parliament, science and societal groups, and simultaneously by TAB's function as an element of public discussion. To this end in-house-assessments are conducted, studies by external scientists and institutes are commissioned, and correspondence workshops are held. The findings, in the form of reports, are passed to the commissioning committee. They can be used by these committees in plenary sessions and for discussions among the working group members of the parliamentary groups, and by the public. They are available to all members of parliament, committees.

Commissions of Enquiry (Enquete-Kommissionen)

1. Functions and tasks: On a motion of at least one quarter of its members, the Bundestag can establish a Commission of Enquiry "for the preparation of decisions on wide-ranging and significant issues". Applications for Commissions of Enquiry stipulate both general tasks and more exactly defined work orders. These commissions investigate the knowledge basis and the practical options for parliament independently of the policies of the executive. New fields of societal development (*e.g.* the effects of the atmospheric warming, or demographic trends) which are difficult to graps, and which require regulation, are the areas usually covered.

The Commissions of Enquiry consist of members of parliament and experts, representatives of interest groups and scientists appointed by the parliamentary political parties. Liaison officers are nominated by the relevant ministries, federal authorities and the Bundesrat in order to guarantee adequate communication with the executive. The parliamentary political groups negotiate which experts are to be appointed, so that in the final instance the power and political arithmetic of the political groups also influence the structure of these commissions.

Commissions of Enquiry are a forum for cooperation between politics and science, integrating scientific expertise services to upgrade the opinion-building process within parliament. The focal task of the study commissions is to take stock of the impacts of technical and economic developments and of potential legal and political measures. To this end, potential developments and regulation problems are being pinpointed and recommendations are made for political decision. The formal goal of the study commission is to prepare interim and final reports, incorporating dissenting opinions. These reports are submitted to the Bundestag for deliberation. Study commissions do not have direct access to parliamentary decision-making processes. They have an advisory function, upstream of decision-making.

2. The instruments of the Commissions of Enquiry: The Commissions of Enquiry harness parliamentary and non-parliamentary expertise in order to acquire information and also tap the knowledge in the working parties in the political parliamentary groups, the parliamentary group support services, the reference and research services, and the ministerial bureaucracy. Wherever necessary, they can also call on inter-authority assistance *(Amtshilfe)*. Every Commission of Enquiry has a secretariat of up to six research staffers on limited contracts. The Bundestag administration, particularly the reference and research services, is responsible for managing the secretariat and for administration. The hearings held by the Commissions of Enquiry and the expert reports commissioned by them are of central importance.

— Public hearings and expert studies: Like the permanent committees, Commissions of Enquiry can also hold public hearings with experts, pressure groups and others. In particular, experts are invited to the hearings that represent institutions or associations which were not taken into account when appointing the commission. It is also possible to hold private hearings. Deliberation is private. Commissions of Enquiry subcontract expert reports, particularly from scientific institutions.

Members of parliament

1. Functions and tasks: The 656 members of the German Bundestag make law and control the government. They represent 328 constituencies and have contested a seat for six political parties, whose policy they represent. By the constitution, they are both representatives of the people and members of a political party.

For individual initiatives such as the tabling of interpellations for oral or written answer, the tabling of motions for debate, and the introduction of private members' bills, the possibilities in the German parliament are negligible. Committees are the dominating structure of the Bundestag. Informal committees are not considered in the Bundestag's Standing Orders, nor are they normal parliamentary practice.

This limits the scope for individual initiatives, because the Standing Orders do foresee initiatives going foward through the parliamentary parties and the committees. An individual MP therefore has to obtain support for his/her issue within the parliamentary group, and get the group to take it up.

2. The instruments available to members of Parliament

— Personal staff: The members of the Bundestag usually employ a personal staff. At the end of 1991, 909 reference and research staff members were employed by members of parliament.

— Parliamentary interpellations: Individual members of parliament can submit interpellations for written or oral answer to the Federal Government *(Einzelfragen zur mündlichen oder schriftlichen Beantwortung)* which are answered in writing within one week or verbally during the weekly interpellation time *(Fragestunde)* in the plenary assembly. In addition, each member of parliament can submit up to four inquiries per month for written reply by the Federal Government.

Parliamentary interpellations *(see above)* to the government are usually made by the opposition parties and their members of parliament. The aim is for the Federal Government, which is nominated by the governing parties, to be obliged to comment on important issues. A political debate can then take place on this basis.

— Reference and Research Service (*Wissenschaftliche Dienste*/W): The Reference and Research Service of the German Bundestag belongs to the general Bundestag administration and has some 2,500 employees. It provides scientific, procedural and organizational support, particularly to individual members of parliament. The working principles of the service are: parliamentary relevance, political neutrality, scientific working methods, appropriate parliamentary presentation, timeliness, uptodateness, and confidentiality.

The Research and Reference Service is divided into four sections: Specialized Research Services 1 and 2, Scientific Documentation and Petitions and Submissions.

• The Specialized Research Services *(Wissen-schaftliche Fachdienste*/WF 1 and WF 2). The WF contains both the committee services with primarily administrative and organizational functions for the different committees of the Bundestag, and also so-called "expert groups" responsible for information acquisition and advisory and consultancy services to the members of parliament. They acquire and organize information and materials for the work of members, and do little research and no scientific analysis themselves. The expert groups thus process information tailored to the needs of those who commissioned it. The areas covered by the nine expert groups are aligned on the division of labour of the parliamentary committee system and thus of the government departments. In 1991 these sections employed a total of 56 experts at the higher civil service, and 36 general staff members.

• Scientific Documentation (*Wissenschaftliche Dokumentation*/WD) is responsible for the Bundestag's library and documentation base. The library contains over 1 million works, and some 12,000 journals and periodicals. Approximately 20,000 articles from 1,600 journals are catalogued each year. Members of parliament can access the parliamentary archives, the Bundestag's own publications and a press cutting service. This work is carried out by some 100 employees.

Members of parliament and the organizational units of the Bundestag can access several bibliographies, facts and texts from some 1,000 data bases including legal and environmental data bases.

- "Petition and Submissions" (Pet) screens the ca 20,000 petitions submitted by citizens each year. The 85 staff members answer these petitions or pass them on to the relevant committees and institutions.

3. Lobbyism and interaction with societal institutions: More than half of the members of the Bundestag hold positions in associations, and two thirds are members of associations. To that extent, MPs are themselves lobbyists. There is talk of an "impressive colouration through associations" *(beeindruckende Verbandsfärbung)* among the parliamentary groups, and some important committees are called "association-islands" for organized interests: *(Verbandsinseln)*.

1,512 associations and their representatives were in 1991 registered on the lobby-list which is published by the President of the Bundestag. The importance of the Bundestag as the partner for such politics is declining: associations and lobbyists are increasingly communicating and bargaining directly with the Executive.

The use of consultation and sources of information: AIDS and genetic engineering/genome analysis

This section lists the parliamentary information instruments used in dealing with the issues of AIDS and genome analysis. No analysis is made of the contents, and no evaluation is made of the relevance, of these instruments.

Plenary assembly

1. Parliamentary interpellations

— Interpellations on AIDS:

- 10th legislative term (1982-1986): no major interpellations, 3 minor ones;

- 11th legislative term (1986-1990): 5 major and 20 minor interpellations;

- 12th legislative term (1990-1994): one major and 4 minor interpellations.

These included in particular the major interpellations on the "Implementation of the resolutions of the German Bundestag on AIDS control of November 13th 1986" raised by the SPD.

— Interpellations on genetic engineering/genome analysis: (1) 10th legislative term (1982-1986): 3 major and 9 minor, (2) 11th legislative term (1986-1990): 5 major and 18 minor, (3) 12th legislative term (1990-1994): no major and 3 minor including particularly a major interpellation on "genetic engineering" from the Green Party.

Parliamentary groups

1. Working parties/groups: As mentioned above, the work in the parliamentary groups is structured very like that of the specialized committees of the Bundestag, and is carried out in working parties/groups, which, in turn are assisted by party support services.

The work units in which the subjects of AIDS and genetic engineering/genome analysis were considered are listed below by way of example:

— Working parties/-groups of the parliamentary parties which considered the subjects of AIDS:

- CDU (Christlich demokratische Union Deutschlands — Christian Democratic Union of Germany): "Health", "Labour and Social Affairs", "Research and Technology", "Internal Affairs", "Family Affairs and Senior Citizens", "Women and Youth";

- SPD (Sozialdemokratische Partei Deutschlands — Social Democratic Party of Germany): "Health", "Labour and the

Social Fabric", "Research and Technology", "Internal Affairs", "Family Affairs and Senior Citizens", "Women and Youth";

- FDP *(Freie demokratische Partei Deutschlands* — Free Democratic Party of Germany): "Labour, Youth, Women, Family, Seniors Citizens and Health Policy", "Internal, Affairs, Legal Affairs, Environment and Sport Policy" and "Educational Policy, Research Policy and Technology Policy".

— Relevant working parties/-groups of the parliamentary parties on genetic engineering/genome analysis:

- CDU: "Health", "Labour and Social Affairs", "Research and Technology", "Family Affairs and Senior Citizens", "Women and Youth";

- SPD: "Health", "Labour and the Social Fabric", "Research and Technology", "Family Affairs and Senior Citizens", "Women and Youth";

- FDP: "Labour, Youth, Women, Family, Senior Citizens and Health Policy", "Internal, Affairs, Legal Affairs, Environment and Sport Policy" and "Educational Policy, Research Policy and Technology Policy".

2. Parliamentary group support services (information not available)

3. Internal parliamentary party hearings, expertise and commentaries (no information available)

Committees

Several permanent committees of the Bundestag are involved in processing legislation on bioethical issues. They hold public hearings but do not publish any reports.

1. Specialized work units

— The following Bundestag committees were involved in the legislative processing of the problem of "AIDS":

- Committee on Family Affairs and Senior Citizens (29 members)
- Committee on Women and Youth (29 members)
- Committee on Health (29 members)
- Committee on Labour and the Social Fabric (37 members)
- Committee on European Community Issue (33 members)
- Committee on Research, Technology and Technology Assessment (35 members)
- Foreign Affairs Committee (41 members)
- Budget Committee (39 members)
- Committee on Internal Affairs (41 members)
- Committee on Legal Affairs (29 members)

— The following Bundestag committees were involved in the legislative processing of the interpellation of genetic engineering/genome analysis:

- Committee on Family Affairs and Senior Citizens (29 members)
- Committee on Women and Youth (29 members)
- Committee on Health (29 members)
- Committee on Labour and the Social Fabric (37 members)
- Committee on European Community Affairs (33 members)
- Committee on Research, Technology and Technology Assessment (35 members)
- Committee on Food, Agriculture and Forestry (35 members)
- Committee on Environment, Nature conservation and nuclear safety (41 members)
- Committee on Economic Affairs (41 members)
- Committee on Economic Cooperation (35 members)
- Committee on Foreign Affairs (41 members)
- Budget Committee (39 members)
- Committee on Internal Affairs (41 members)
- Committee on Legal Issues (29 members)

2. Public hearings

— Hearings on AIDS: The committee for Youth, Family,

Women and Health held a public hearing on 19th March 1986 on:

- "Combatting the acquired immune deficiency syndrome (AIDS)" and
- "Measures to control AIDS". This hearing lead to the establishment of a study commission.

The Committee on Health held a public hearing on 12th June 1991 on:

- "AIDS in the new federal states and Eastern European countries"

and on 25th September 1991 on:
- "Conclusions from the report of the study commission on AIDS for an effective AIDS control policy in the former federal states".

— Hearings on genetic engineering/genome analysis: The committee on legal issues held a public hearing on 3rd February 1988 on the study commission's report:
- "Opportunities and risks of genetic engineering".

On 24th February 1988, the committee for Youth, Family, Women and Health Affairs together with the Committee for Labour and the Social Fabric and the Committee on Research and Technology held a public hearing on the study commission's report.
- "Opportunities and risks of genetic engineering", specifically covering issues of genome analysis of employees.

On the same day, together with the Committee for Research and Technology, it held a further public hearing on the study commission's report.
- "Opportunities and risks of genetic engineering", specifically covering the issues of prenatal diagnostics.

The Committee for Youth, Family, Women and Health held a public hearing from 17th to 19th January 1990 on:
- "The draft bill to regulate genetic engineering issues"

The Committee for Research and Technology held a public hearing on 2nd March 1988 on:
- "The release of genetically manipulated organisms".

3. The Technology Assessment Unit (TAB): On behalf of the Federal Parliamentary Committee for Research, Technology and Technology Assessment, TAB commenced a TA project on genome analysis in June 1991.

Several studies were commissioned from external experts on the following subject:

— present state and prospects of genome analysis;
— application prospects and regulation potentials for genome analysis in the world of work;
— prospects of applying genome analysis in the fields of human genetics, insurance, penal and civil processes and the pertinent potential for regulation;
— the image of "biotechnological safety" and "genome analysis" in the German daily press (1988-1990);
— one legal and one scientific study.

TAB held two workshops with members of parliament and experts (TAB info N° 9). A public poll was conducted.

— TAB publications:

- Genetic engineering and genome analysis in the public's view (TAB discussion paper N° 3).
- The image of "biological safety" and "genome analysis" in the German daily press (1988-1990) (TAB discussion paper N° 2).
- Status and prospects of using genetic tests (preli-minary findings from the TA project "genome analysis").

The final report on the "genome analysis" project was presented in June 1993 and published in October 1993.

Commissions of Enquiry (Enquete-Kommissionen)

1. Composition and functioning: There are no special advisers on bioethical issues at the Bundestag. However, specialist were employed on limited-term contracts in the Secretariat for the purposes of the Commissions of Enquiry on AIDS and Genetic Engineering.

— AIDS: On 8th May 1987 the German Bundestag resolve to establish a Commission of Enquiry on "the risks of AIDS and effective ways of containing them". The 17 members of the commission comprised nine members of parliament nominated in accordance with the strength of the political parties and eight external experts from clinics, scientific institutes, the office of the Federal Attorney, and a self-help organisation. The secretariat of the study commission consisted of the director, and on average, four reference and research and five general staff members.

In all, the Commission of Enquiry held a total of 78 mostly full day commission meetings.

— Genetic engineering/genome analysis: The Commission of Enquiry on "Opportunities and risks of genetic engineering" was established on 14th August 1984 and completed its work with the submission of a final report in December 1986. The commission consisted of nine members of parliament nominated in accordance with parliamentary party strengths and eight external experts — for example from medicine, biology and theology, representatives of trade unions and the pharmaceutical industry. A reference and research secretariat was established with six reference and three research staff.

The study commission was broken down into six reporting/working groups including working group IV on health, working group V on genetic analysis and working group VI on gene therapy.

The Commission of Enquiry held 55 commission meetings and 46 working group meetings.

2. Hearings and commissioned studies

— AIDS: 21 one or two-day public hearings were held, to which a total of 230 external experts were invited.

Seven studies were contracted out to external scientists and institutes, several scientific congresses and clinics were visited in Germany and abroad, and a study trip made to Uganda and Rwanda.

A first interim report was submitted on 16th June 1988 (BT-Doc. 11/2495) which was debated in the plenary session on 27th October 1988. The final report was presented on 26th May 1990 (11/7200) and debated in the plenary session of parliament on 28th February 1991.

— Genetic engineering/genome analysis: 18 hearings were held, four of which were open to the public and involved external expertise. For example, the public hearing covered the following issues: "genetic counselling and the genetic analysis of human beings", "the scientific prerequisites for gene-technological operations on human beings", and the genetic analysis of workers.

The individual working groups of the study commission held a further 3 hearings. The study commission commissioned four expert reports and numerous written studies from external persons and organizations. The commission made a study trip to Japan and its members attended numerous conferences and visited institutes and industrial companies.

The final report of the study commission was submitted on 19th January 1987 and subsequently debated in plenary. It contains ca 200 individual recommendations. At the end of 1990, the Federal Government presented another report (BT Doc. 11/8520) about the way to apply the resolutions of the Bundestag on the original report. This second report was debated in plenary on 28th February 1991.

Members of Parliament

1. Parliamentary interpellations:

— Individual enquiries on AIDS

- 10th legislative term (1982-1986): 26 written and 7 oral interpellations;
- 11th legislative term (1986-1990): 55 written and 16 oral interpellations;
- 12th legislative term (1990-1994): 9 written and 3 oral interpellations.

— Individual enquiries on genetic engineering

- 10th legislative term (1982-1986): 9 written and 6 oral interpellations;
- 11th legislative term (1986-1990): 29 written and 5 oral interpellations;
- 12th legislative term (1990-1994): no written and 3 oral interpellations.

2. Reference and Research services

The following units of the Reference and Research Services sub-section (WFD 2) are particularly relevant to AIDS and genetic engineering/genome analysis:

- VI: Labour and Social Issues;
- VII: Civil, penal and procedural law, environmental protection law, regional planning, construction, urban development;
- VIII: Research, Technology, Education and Science, Environment, Nature Protection, Reactor Safety;
- IX: Health, Family and Senior Citizens, Women and Youth.

— The following general papers on AIDS were prepared for members of parliament by the Scientific Documentation subsection (WD):

- Documentation: "AIDS — basic medical information in keywords" 1987 (21 pages);

- Bibliography: "AIDS, acquired immune deficiency syndrome" (1987);
- Bibliography: "AIDS, acquired immune deficiency syndrome" (1989).

- Reports on the following subjects: legal regulations in the Federal Republic relevant to AIDS; local government measures against AIDS; penal problems in introducing substitution programs for HIV positive drug addicts; legal problems and regulation potentials for voluntary HIV testing in medical examinations for job seekers; AIDS — present status of prevention, diagnosis and therapy, and the attendant social problems; penal regulations in the event of infection by HIV infected persons; legality and possible legal basis for pinpointing AIDS-infected persons in the police information system (INPOL); the disease AIDS, with particular reference to the legal problems; the situation of young people as regards family planning, AIDS and abortion in the former USSR.

— The "Scientific Documentation" subsection also prepared the following general documentation for members of parliament on subject of genetic engineering/genome analysis:

- "Genome analysis and gene therapy" and
- "Genetic degradation".

The library holds 35 journals that are pertinent to AIDS and genetic testing.

The members and the Bundestag's services have access to some 1,000 external databases. The Bundestag library uses 9 databases for AIDS and 13 for genetic testing.

Notes on the current situation in Germany

There are, at the moment, neither general nor special explicit statutory provisions on the admissibility, the procedure and the utilization of the results of genetic testing/screening. Therefore the general legal provisions and rules of the German legal system have to be applied (*e.g.* Civil Code, Criminal Code, Federal Data Protection Act).

On a voluntary basis, prenatal diagnoses by genetic analysis are admissible. Postnatal diagnoses are also subject to the individual right of self-determination. A general and comprehensive genetic analysis prescribed by the state as part of public health policy would be unlawful.

Concerning the goals of prevention of and protection from AIDS, there are today no explicit or specific statutory provisions. Therefore the relevant rules and provisions of current laws *(e.g.* the Federal Epidemics Act — *Bundesseuchengesetz)* have to be applied.

Annexe 1

Overview of the working and consultative (advisory) structures on different levels at the German Bundestag

Institutional level	Information instruments
Plenary Assembly *(Plenum)*	Parliamentary interpellation
Parliamentary political groups *(Fraktionen)*	The parliamentary group services studies and comments
Permanent committees *(Fachausschüsse)*	Comments and opinions Hearings Technology Assessment Unit (TAB)
Commissions of Enquiry *(Enquete-Kommissionen)*	Public hearings and expert studies
Members of Parliament *(Abgeordnete)*	Personal staff member Parliamentary interpellations Reference and Research Service (WD)

Annexe 2

External experts of the two Commissions of Enquiry on AIDS and Genome analysis/genetic engineering

a) External experts of the Commission of Enquiry *(Enquete-Kommission)* on « AIDS » :

1. Sophinette Becker (psychologist), Abteilung für Sexualwissenschaft, Klinikum der Johann-Wolfgang-Goethe-Universität, Frankfurt/M.
2. Manfred Bruns, Bundesanwalt beim Bundesgerichtshof.
3. Prof, Dr. Hans-Ullrich Gallwas, Institut für Politik und Öffentliches Recht, Ludwig-Maximilian-Universität, München.
4. Dieter Riehl, Deutsche AIDS-Hilfe e.V., Hannover.
5. Dr, Rolf Rosenbrock, Wissenschaftszentrum, Berlin.
6. Prof. Dr. Wolfgang Spann, Vorstand des Instituts für Rechtsmedizin, Ludwig-Maximilian-Universität, München.
7. Prof. Dr. Wolfgang Stille, Zentrum für Innere Medizin, Johann-Wolfgang-Goethe-Universität, Frankfurt/M.
8. Prof. Dr. Nepomuk Zöllner, Vorstand der Medizinischen Poliklinik, Ludwig-Maximilian-Universität, München.

b) External experts of the Commission of Enquiry *(Enquete-Komission)* on « Opportunities and risks of gene technology » :

1. Dr. Wolfgang van den Daele (Wissenschaftsforschung), Universität Bielefeld.
2. Prof. Dr. Erwin Deutsch (Recht), Universität Göttingen.
3. Prof. Dr. med. Gisela Nass-Hennig (Molekulare Genetik), Universität Freiburg.
4. Dr. med. Erwin Odenbach (Bundesärztekammer), Köln.
5. Prof. Dr. Hans-Jürgen Quadbeck-Seeger (Industrie), BASF AG Ludwigshafen.
6. Prof. Dr. Johannes Reiter (Moraltheologe), Universität Mainz.
7. Jürgen Walter (Deutscher Gewerkschaftsbund), IG Chemie-Papier-Keramik Hannover.
8. Prof. Dr. Ernst-Ludwig Winnacker (Biochemie), Universität München.

The means of information available to the Hellenic Chamber of Deputies on matters of bioethics

STEPHANOS I. KOUTSOUBINAS[1]

A preliminary remark

The bioethical debate in Greece is still at an embryonic stage. Public opinion, ill or little informed, seems indifferent and the press pays little attention. Opinion polls show that the Greeks are among the most enthusiastic for the application of evolving technologies both to the food industry and to medicine, without worrying too much about possible bad consequences, predictable or unpredictable. In the university context, debate has just started; in Greek industry, which, to a large measure, is traditional, it is not thought that the issues raised by biotechnology need dealing with or regulating with any urgency.

This situation is reflected, as one might expect, in that mirror of society that a Chamber of representatives elected by the people is supposed to be. Thus, there does not exist, for the moment, any special law dealing with bioethical problems; where

---

1. From the Research Department of the Hellenic Parliament.

conflicts emerge, they are resolved on the basis of existing general legislation by way of the civil or the penal code[2].

Nor has any general discussion yet taken place in the Chamber of Deputies, either in plenary session or in special Committee (with the notable exception of questions of AIDS); nor has any report been prepared and presented to the Chamber by the Deputies or by the services of he Chamber on the subject of bioethics.

What follows, consequently, does not describe "how information about the progress and potentialities of the revolution in human microbiology, and its actual and potential ethical and social effects, is acquired and handled"[3] by the Greek Chamber of Deputies, but how this could happen in the future, which surely will not be long delayed, in accordance with established parliamentary procedure and with parliamentary reality in Greece.

A general glance

Since 1975, the Greek political system has been that of a parliamentary republic. There is only one legislative Chamber, which is traditionally called the Vouli; it is composed of 300 deputies and is completely renewed every four years. The tripartite separation of the powers of the State is solemnly affirmed in the Constitution. The provisions of the constitution norms take precedence over the other rules composing the Greek juridical order, a precedence which it is the duty of all the judicial instances of the country to take account of.

---

2. Recently, a Commission of experts has been set up to prepare a draft law concerning the problems raised by medically assisted procreation. This will be the first time that a discussion on bioethics has taken place in the Chamber of Deputies.
3. Lord Kennet, *The interface between Bioethics and Parliaments in five European Community States*, Introduction to Parliaments and screening for HIV and genetic disease.

The President of the Chamber of Deputies is elected by the whole legislature. His powers, and also political practicality, make the President's role closer to the Continental model than to that of the British Speaker.

The Government, elected and supported by a Parliamentary majority following a vote of confidence, is usually unitary. Since 1975, coalition governments have been rare; the electoral system of adjusted proportional representation does not favour it. The Prime Minister is, in effect, the strong man of the regime.

The political parties, recognized by the Constitution not only as performers in the electoral game, but also as permanent factors in all political life, are quite strongly structured. The personal power of the leader of a party is considerable and party discipline, especially at the moment of the voting, is of iron. It is for this reason that initiatives coming from the Deputies themselves are relatively rare, and they are almost always conditioned and guided by the party to which the Deputy belongs.

Legislative initiative belongs concurrently to the Chamber of Deputies and to the Government. In practice, it is effectively exercised only by the Government; among some 2200 laws which have been voted on since 1975, only two or three have been of parliamentary origin, and they concern subjects of minor importance.

The internal resources of the Chamber of Deputies

The internal services of the Chamber

Among the internal services of the Chamber, the Library and the Direction of Studies are able to produce information and studies on bioethical questions for the Deputies.

— The Library of the Chamber of Deputies, founded in 1845, is today among the richest parliamentary libraries in the world. Its priority orientation is towards politics, human and social sciences, and it continues to improve its collections. There is a complete series of the Greek Official Journal and of the community's official documents, as well as a large number of the Official Journals of the principal European countries. There is no special section for publications dealing with bioethics or bioetchnology.

— The research department was created in 1989. It consists of two sections, one for the technical and juridical application of bills, and the other for parliamentary studies and research. Each section consists of seven researchers, most of them graduates from the Hellenic Law Faculties. Its includes remit "scientific assistance in comparative law and technical and juridical assistance of the Chamber in the exercise of its legislative work and in its general parliamentary work". Each Deputy has the right to request information and advice (especially in juridical matters), which the Department must treat "using as sole criterion the general principals and rules of the science".

— There are also the Deputies' assistants. Each Deputy has effectively the right to recruit a limited number of assistants (who are paid by the Chamber) to assist the Deputy in his or her parliamentary activities.

Parliamentary debates

Discussion relating to bioethical problems can take place in the Chamber of Deputies: independently of a bill, in connection with a bill, in connection with parliamentary control.

1. Independently of a bill

— Various informal committees are set up by the deputies. They are not established by the rules of the Chamber and can be freely organized on any subject, and can be permanent or ad-hoc (for instance the different Greek friendship committees with other countries). Their members are not always exclusively parliamentarians and, unlike the other committees of the Chamber, their memberhip needs not be proportional to that of the parliamentary groups; most groups are represented on them, but this is not always the case. These committees, whose activities are carried out both inside and outside the Chamber, can become vehicles of information for the Chamber on society's concerns, and can sensitize the parliamentary machine to new situations.

— In a more organized and more political context, the Chamber itself may decide, at the suggestion of the Government or of the chairmen of parliamentary groups, to set up special Committees for the study of matters of general interest: the most recent is on the reform of the penal system, which reported in July 1994.

These special Committees are entirely composed of deputies (though assisted in their work by specialists), proportionally to the strength of the different parliamentary groups in the Chamber. They have a precise role (described in the Chamber's resolution which institutes them) and a period within which their proposals must be submitted.

The special Committes summon expert witnesses, make visits, and conduct various investigations (however without having the competence of the commissions of inquiry), study the relative documentation and, eventually, produce a report with information and proposals. Minority opinions are included in this report, which is consultative in character, and submitted to the Government and to the Chamber of Deputies. Often enough, at the initiative of either the Government or the opposition, a general debate takes place in the Chamber on these reports, and occasionally, legislative changes follow.

— It is possible for the Chamber of Deputies itself, *via* its President, to institute a sort of ad hoc expert committee for the study of a particular problem and the submission of a report or of advice. But this is an unusual practice.

2. In connection with a bill

Government Bills are drafted by the relevant ministries. Each bill is required to be accompanied by a statement of purpose, which is intended to provide the necessary elements of information to justify the proposals.

The bill is first examined by the competent permanent parliamentary committee. There are six permanent committees (cultural affairs, national defence and foreign affairs, finance, social affairs, administration of public order and justice, and lastly production and trade: a committee on European affairs has recently been added to them). The composition of these Committees reflects the composition of the Chamber as a whole.

The sessions of the permanent committees at the initial discussion on the principle of the bill are public. At this stage, the Committees may question extra-parliamentary persons who are capable of clarifying the Committee's members on special or technical subjects.

At the end of the examination of each bill (whether government or parliamentary in origin), the competent Committee having voted the same with any amendments, it is transmitted to the plenary assembly of the Chamber for the next stages of the legislative procedure.

In parallel with the work of the committee, the bill is examined by the relevant section of the Research Department. The report of the latter, strictly juridical and with no reference to any of the political implications of the proposals, is also submitted to the President of the Chamber and distributed to all the deputies before the beginning of debates.

The debate in the plenary Assembly takes place as in all other European parliaments; the discussion is well organized; only deputies (and Ministers) may speak, bill is voted once on the principle, now article by article, now on the whole. There is no procedure for a blocking vote in Greece.

One may remark that the Standing Orders of the Chamber ensure, in principle, that all means are available for the information of the deputies on scientific, social or ethical issues of the questions debated in the Chamber. The special committees, the expert committees, the questioning of extra-parliamentary persons, and the reports of the Research Department are so many links of communication carrying the necessary information to the legislative act. The system has functioned pretty well so far for other subjects, and there is nothing to prevent it functioning equally well in the future, when the great issues of bioethics and biotechnology come to be debated.

3. In connection with parliamentary control

— The means of parliamentary control in Greek constitutional law are reports, questions, requests for documents, interpellations, and discussions preceding the order of the day. All these means, exclusively exercised by the Deputies, can bring to the knowledge of the Chamber, in an official manner, information on the social aspects of bioethical questions, and on the people's state of mind about them.

— The Chamber of Deputies may also set up through its members, Committees of Inquiry, to examine subjects of special public interest. The initiative for setting up these committees (unlike the special committees already mentioned) can only be taken in Parliament. They have the powers of a court of law. They reach reasoned conclusions which must also state the views of the minority, and they submit them to the Chamber. On a proposal supported by one-fifth of the total number of Deputies, these conclusions can be placed on the Order Paper and debated in plenary Assembly.

Sources external to the Parliament

The Church

Being the church of the dominant religion in Greece, the Greek Orthodox Church has a particular status among the other churches, and is not completely separate from the State, yet there is no officially established line of communication between it and the Chamber of Deputies. The opinion of the Church is always requested when religious affairs or the internal organization of ecclesiastical life are discussed. It is of course evident that, in relation to other questions, the Church's points of view are taken up and expressed in the Chamber by Deputies. (Ecclesiastics may not be Deputies).

In any case, the Greek Church has not yet adopted an official position on any bioethical proposition, except for euthanasia, which it rigorously condemns.

The Athens Academy and the Universities

There is no direct or long term co-operation between the Chamber of Deputies and these institutions. As has been seen earlier, the members of the Academy and the universities are quite frequently invited by the Chamber, though in their personal capacity, to participate in the various expert committees and to submit their own scientific advice.

There is no established interaction between public opinion and the Chamber of Deputies in Greece (on the model, for example, of the Danish system of Consensus Conferences).

Bioethical information in the Irish Parliament

VERONA NI BHROINN[1]

Ireland is a parliamentary democracy. The sole power of making laws is vested in Parliament which consists of two Houses: the House of Representatives (Dáil Éireann) and the Senate (Seanad Éireann). Under the Constitution, the executive power of the State shall be exercised by or under the authority of the Government whose policy and administration may be examined and criticized in both Houses. However, under the Constitution, the Government is responsible to the Dáil alone.

Parliamentary procedure

For the purposes of this survey, it is the procedure in Dáil Éireann, whose Members are directly elected by universal suffrage, which is principally described. The Constitution devolves on each House the power to make its own rules and Standing Orders and these are supplemented by Sessional Orders (Orders that amend or set aside a Standing Order for a specified period), *ad hoc* orders, resolutions and precedent (Mr. Speaker's rulings).

---

1. Public Relations Officer of the Parliament.

There are four main procedural ways in which members may elicit information in Dáil Éirean:

— questions,
— bills,
— estimates,
— motions.

Questions

Standing Orders of Dáil Éireann allow members to address questions to a member of the Government about "public affairs connected with his/her Department on matters of public administration for which he/she is officially responsible". There are two categories of parliamentary questions, viz. oral questions, in respect of which a member may ask supplementary questions, at the discretion of the Chair, while replies to written questions are printed in the official report of each day's proceedings. Additionally, a private notice question which the Ceann Comhairle (Mr. Speaker) deems related to a matter of urgent public importance may be permitted on short notice. Members may also raise matters of administration relating to a minister's department on the motion for the daily adjournment of the House. It is likely that questions regarding screening for HIV and genetic disease would be within the responsibility of the Minister of Health.

Bills

At the appropriate stages of the passage of a Government Bill through the legislative process, members may raise policy issues and table relevant amendments and may also, subject to certain criteria, publish their own bills which are generally debated in Private Members Time, *i.e.* a time specifically allocated under Standing Orders for such business.

Estimates

Again it is open to members, either in the House or in Committee *(see below)* to raise issues on the annual estimates of expenditure for each Government Department.

Motions

It is open to any member to table a motion on any subject and such motions would normally be debated in Private Members Time. Members may also contribute to debates on Government business when such business is brought before the Dáil by way of motion.

Under Standing Orders, a member may move the adjournment of the Houses for the purpose of debating "a specific and important matter of public interest requiring urgent consideration". If the request is permitted by the Ceann Comhairle and receives the support of at least 12 members, the matter is discussed in the last one and a half hours of the sitting, or as the Dáil may order.

Legislative Committees in Parliament

The Houses of the Oireachtas also conduct some of their proceedings through a system of parliamentary committees. While Parliament has always had the power to appoint special, select or joint committees to deal with specific stages of bills, the past twelve months have seen the establishment of new sessional legislative committees each of which has the responsibility, inter alia, for processing bills and examining departmental estimates under five main categories of Parliamentary business:

— social affairs,
— finance and general affairs,
— enterprise and economic strategy,
— legislation and security,
— foreign affairs.

N°s 1,2,3, and 4 are Dáil Committees. N° 5 is a Joint Committee of both Houses.

These new committees have parallel terms of reference and, in the context of this survey, the Select Committee on Social Affairs considers, inter alia, matters relating to social welfare, health, education and equality.

Each committee makes an annual report to Dáil Éireann which details the work carried out, work in progress and the attendance and voting records at meetings of the Committee. Subject to the consent of the Minister of Finance, each Committee has power to engage the services of persons with specialist or technical knowledge to assist it or any of its subcommittees in their consideration of matters. Such Committees may also invite submissions in writing from interested persons or bodies. Members other than members of the committee may also attend and participate in such meetings, but without having voting rights.

Recent years have seen progress in making the work of Parliament more transparent and relevant to the electorate. In this regard, Dáil reform is an ongoing process and, at present, initiatives in the area of compellability of witnesses before committees are being addressed.

Tribunals of inquiry

While recourse to such inquiries is rare, tribunals of inquiry are set up by resolution of Parliament and can make recommendations. The establishment of such inquiries generally reflects the absolute priority accorded to the Tribunal by Parliament to examine in the most open, authoritative, independent and comprehensive manner available under statute, the issues under referral. The most recent Tribunal of Inquiry was the "Tribunal of Inquiry into The Beef Processing Industry", which was established pursuant to resolutions of both Houses in May 1991, and which made many recommendations in its report.

Information and research service for members

The Oireachtas Library provides an information and research service for members of both Houses and holds information on biomedical ethics including UK parliamentary papers, EU documentation and other official publications.

While the Library does not subscribe to journals dealing specifically with bioethical issues, it holds several titles relating to health and medicine. When a member requests information dealing with scientific and technological subjects, newspaper and journal articles can be retrieved from the *FT Profile* database and the Library can also access the resources of other libraries and organizations (*e.g.* Government Departments, research organizations) as well as those of foreign parliaments. In addition, it currently subscribes to the information services offered by Trinity College Library (University of Dublin) and by Radio Telefís Éireann (the national broadcasting station) which undertake research on its behalf (*e.g.* by carrying out on-line speeches, supplying relevant journal articles).

Formal parliamentary links with churches/academic institutions

The Constitution of Ireland guarantees not to endow any religion. As a result of the constitutional separation of Church and State, there are no formal established parliamentary links with the Churches, but it would be true that Church and State take cognizance of each other's positions. In relation to academic institutions, the constitutions provides for the election of six members to the Senate to be made by the university constituencies of the National University of Ireland (3) and the University of Dublin (Trinity College) (3). The electorate for these constituencies comprises graduates of these institutions.

Regulation of lobbyists

A formal lobbying system does not operate in the Irish Parliamentary system but any member of the public or public interest group seeking information regarding a specific subject, is free to contact party members who, in turn, can avail themselves of parliamentary procedure to address the issues. Moreover, individuals and/or groups may often request a politician or political group to make representations on their behalf.

Legislation (affecting issues appertaining to AIDS)

— The Health (Family Planning) (Amendment) Act, 1993. This Act deregulated the supply of condoms in Ireland — an initiative that ensures that condoms are accessible to persons who wish to practise safe sex.

— The Criminal Law (Sexual Offences) Act, 1993. This Act decriminalised homosexual acts between consenting male adults over 17 years of age.

The Department of Health — AIDS/HIV prevention and education initiatives

The Department of Health has statutory responsibility for all health issues. While screening for HIV and genetic disease is not at present regulated by statute, the Department of Health has taken, and funded, certain on-going initiatives in these areas.

In recent years a multimedia campaign was put in place to raise public awareness about HIV and AIDS and this ongoing campaign involves radio, television and newspaper advertisements. Other measures include AIDS education resource materials for second level schools, an educational video, convenience advertising and financial support for a wide number of specialist voluntary AIDS service organizations.

Screening for HIV

Since 1985, a programme for voluntary linked HIV testing has been in operation. As a result of recommendations made by the National AIDS Strategy Committee, which is a non-statutory but Government funded organization, the Department of Health has now extended the programme through unlinked anonymous HIV Surveillance. The Report of the National AIDS Strategy Committee is the basis for an integrated and coordinated strategy in this area. The Committee's terms of reference are: "To keep under review programmes and services relating to AIDS and HIV, to monitor the implementation of the AIDS Strategy to ensure that it is appropriate and responsive to the evolving epidemiology of the disease and to make recommendations to Government, as appropriate, about the Strategy."

Screening for genetic disease

July 1994 saw the appointment, in the public domain, of the first genetic consultant in the State and women carrying foetuses with chromosomal abnormalities and genetic defects are counselled on a non-directive basis. In 1992, the Constitution of Ireland was amended following a referendum in favour of providing a right to information on abortion, and legislation is currently being prepared to give effect to that constitutional right.

Aids related motions discussed in private members' time

— 26 April 1989 — Trust fund for Aids infected HIV positive haemophiliacs and general policy regarding all Aids sufferers.

— 28 November 1990 — National Aids Plan.

Bioethics in the Italian Parliament

STEFANO RODOTA[1]

The Italian Parliament has not shown any particular interest in the various questions which are grouped under the term "bioethics". No evidence has been heard and no new committees have been created: there is thus no basic documentation comparable to that which has been produced by other parliaments and which has contributed to fuller information and more rational debate among the public. For internal purposes only, and therefore without any external circulation, the Research Department of the Senate has decided to collect and translate the most important legislative texts and judicial judgements from other countries.

It is also interesting to note that the Chamber of Deputies has not thought it necessary to set up an office on the model of the US Office of Technology Assessment, despite the fact that since the mid eighties the setting up of such an office has been formally requested by the leaders of all the party groups, and has been unanimously approved.

---

1. Professor of Jurisprudence in the University of Rome. Member of Parliament.

Tenth Legislature (1987-1992)

In the course of the Tenth Legislature (of the Republic: 1987-92), the most important events were as follows:

— The approval of the Law of 5 June 1990 on the HIV syndrome, which is of particular interest because it provides strong guarantees of privacy. But this privacy provision was later limited by another law of 1990 providing for the possibility of screening applicants for enrolment in the Police for HIV, the results of such tests to be known only to particular services. The protection of privacy was later further limited by a decision of the Constitutional Court in 1994 which admitted the possibility of screening for reasons of general interest.

— The passing of the Law of 4 May 1990 which regulates the transfusion of human blood and plasma products.

— A general debate in the Chamber of Deputies which passed a motion demanding, among other things, a moratorium on experimentation in the biotechnology sector. This moratorium has never been applied.

— The laying of various proposals for the constitution of a Parliamentary Committee of inquiry on biotechnology. The proposals were discussed in the Constitutional Affairs Committee of the Chamber, but were not approved.

— The laying of numerous bills about artificial insemination, transplants and the definition of death. None of these bills was approved.

During this legislature, the National Bioethical Committee was founded. Parliament, however, had nothing to do with its foundation, since it is purely nominated by the Government.

Eleventh Legislature (1992-1994)

In the course of the eleventh Legislature (1992-94), the most important events were the following:

— The Law of 12 December 1993 which effected major reforms in the criteria for the definition of death: Article 1 provides that death should be identified by the irreversible cessation of all brain functions.

— A law on cornea transplants which introduced the principle of the agreement of the donor or members of his or her family.

— A debate in the Chamber of Deputies on 29 and 30 June 1993 on bioethics, which passed a rather generic motion.

— Five bills about artificial insemination and two about the protection of the human embryo were laid. They strongly reflected the differing "ideological" positions present in the Italian Parliament. The bills presented by the Christian Democrats and the Right were based above all on the protection of the embryo and had a pronounced anti-abortion purpose; as for the technologies of reproduction, they tended towards prohibition. The other bills admitted the possibility of access to reproductive technology by single and non-sterile women, and aimed particularly to fill two serious gaps in Italian law: the lack of any supervision for the centres where these treatments are done, and the possibility of the disaffiliation of a son by a man who has agreed to the impregnation of his wife or partner with the sperm of a donor. None of these bills even reached the stage of preliminary examination.

— Fourteen bills were laid about transplants (especially of the cornea), both between living people and from corpses.

During the Twelfth Legislature, which began in April 1994, there has been a particular interest in bioethics. This novelty, besides marking an increase in cultural maturity, can be explained by two things: on the one hand, the strong public feeling about cases such as the so-called "granny mums", and, on the other, the judgement of the Court at Cremona which permitted a father, who had consented to the impregnation of his wife with the sperm of a donor, to disaffiliate his son; and on the other hand the strongly political values assumed by the main themes of bioethics, which some hope to use to obtain the support of Catholic electors (and of the Church) after the disappearance of the traditional Catholic party, Christian Democracy.

Many parliamentary questions have been asked, calling for explanations of certain cases of clinical experimentation on persons and animals, the removal of organs, the acquisition of human blood abroad, and the conditions of AIDS sufferers in prison. On this last question, many bills have also been presented.

Two bills have also been presented on clinical experiments on persons, four on transplants, and four on reproductive technologies. None of these has got as far as initial examination.

Biotechnology and the Luxembourg Parliament[1]

FRANCINE COCARD[2]

The Special Genetics Committee (CSG) of the Luxembourg Parliament was constituted in July 1990, and its aim was to prepare a public debate about biotechnology. Parliament found it necessary to constitute this committee following the adoption by the European Council in April 1990, of directives 90/219 and 90/220 on genetically modified organisms.

A debate on biotechnology in the Luxembourg Parliament took place on 20 November 1991. During its preparatory work, the Committee inquired about the laws and legislative work existing in the neighbouring countries of Belgium, France and Germany. It set up a library with medical dictionaries and details of research done mainly in France and Germany. The members of the Committee had meetings with representatives of all

---

1. The Parliament of Luxembourg (the Chamber of Deputies) shares legislative power with the Grand Duke. The constitution assigns it decisive power in financial matters, and the right to supervise the actions of the Government. In international affairs, the consent of the Chamber is required before a treaty can come into effect on the territory of the Grand-Duchy.
  The Chamber of Deputies is a single House, and its 60 members represent five parties. Seats in the Parliament are allocated according to proportional representation, on the principle of the smallest electoral quota. They are spread over the different lists of candidates proportionally to the number of votes cast for them.
2. Clerk of Committees.

the ministries concerned with biotechnology, such as the departments of Health, the Environment, Agriculture, Economics, the Family, Justice and Employment.

The Committee heard a presentation by the president of the National Consultative Committee for Ethics (the "Commission Consultative Nationale d'Éthique"). It also had discussions with representatives of the only medical laboratory then using genetically modified micro-organisms, and with lawyers specializing in the legal and ethical aspects of biotechnology.

A second debate about biotechnology took place in October 1992, on the patenting biotechnological "inventions". The Committee's mandate had been extended to prepare this debate as well, and it analysed existing texts produced by the European Commission. It inquired about the economic and legal character of patents.

Both debates were preceded by the publication of two reports written by the Parliamentary Committee, and, in both debates, the Parliament's message to the Government was clear: it recommended extreme care whenever products containing biotechnologically modified substances were put on the market, and the same caution where a company sought permission to establish a plant, or where the question was whether to patent a biologically modified part of the human body.

In February 1994, for ethical reasons, Luxembourg voted against the "Common Position" of the European Council on the patenting of biotechnological "inventions".

In 1993-94, the CSG analysed the way in which the two European Directives were to be implemented in Luxembourgish law. It also held a meeting on the cloning of human embryos.

The Luxembourg Parliament does not have a specialized staff to deal with questions of biotechnology; and one ordinary member of staff is in charge of work for the special Committee. Members of Parliament may consult the information, documentation and reports available in the Committee's library.

The legislative procedure in Luxembourg ensures that bills presented by the Government are examined by the "Chambres Professionelles" and by other representative bodies of the professions. The Committee thus attends to a broad spectrum of opinion. All notes upon, criticisms of, or reactions to biotechnology sent to Parliament by any association, organization, or private person interested in the matter, are transmitted to the Committee by the President of the Parliament.

In general, the members of Parliament follow the Committee in stressing caution, even in the face of potential economic gain. And so far, the members of Parliament have not expressed any discontent with the quantity of information available, or with the relations with the Government and non-governmental organizations.

Providing the Netherlands Parliament with information on normative aspects of testing and screening for HIV and genetic diseases [1]

G.M.W.R. DE WERT [2], I. RAVENSCHLAG [2], M.A.M. DE WACHTER [2]

Stating the problem and its background

The potential for screening and testing is ever increasing. Not only within health care but also on the job market and in the context of social services such as insurance, screening and testing become more and more important. The fields of AIDS and genetics raise numerous issues for screening and testing.

The Netherlands is a constitutional monarchy. Its Parliament contains two Chambers. The "Second Chamber" is directly elected by proportional representation. There are many political parties. Government is represented in the Second Chamber by a coalition of parties. Individual members of the government cannot be members of the Second Chamber. The "First Chamber" consists of members indirectly elected by the Provincial States. The First Chamber checks legislation after it has been approved by the Second Chamber. It does, however, have

---
1. The authors wish to thank the numerous informants of many organizations named in this report, who were helpful in providing information.
2. From the Institute for Bioethics, Maastricht.

less rights than the Second Chamber. For example, the First Chamber has no right to amend, it can only say "yes" or "no" to decisions taken by the Second Chamber.

Sooner or later, Parliament must decide whether to regulate HIV and genetic screening. Such decisions are complex because of the manifold social, ethical, and legal implications, and well informed decision making is of the greatest importance. The question which occasioned this report was: how does the Dutch Parliament inquire about the social, ethical, and legal issues of screening and testing in the fields of genetics and of HIV-infection?

In this report we use a rather wide definition of screening and testing. Screening: we take it to be the testing of an asymptomatic population in order to identify people who may be HIV infected (HIV screening), and people who may possess a particular genotype (genetic screening).

Our enquiry followed two paths: the stream of available information offered to Parliament, on the one hand, and the stream of information which, in actual fact, was requested by members of Parliament on the other. Both approaches ought to offer a fair picture of what information did reach the members of Parliament.

Scope and goals of this report

The primary goal of this report is to draw a picture of the current stream of information which may reach the Dutch Parliamentarian about the fields of screening and testing for genetic deviations and for HIV infection. Our first task was to make a descriptive inventory. But we decided not to include the debate on the registration and use of hereditary information (genetic registers), nor issues concerning cell banks. Similarly, we omitted HIV-testing of the donors of blood, organs and gametes. Forensic applications of screening and testing, on the other hand, though not intended to discover genetic disease but only to establish a similarity between two samples, seemed to be of such immediate interest that we felt it necessary to include them.

Non-parliamentary bodies

In the Netherlands, a great many independent committees inform Parliament. In this section, we shall name such instances and mention the reports they have provided over the recent past in the areas of HIVST (HIV screening and testing) and GDST (genetic disease screening and testing).

The Council of State (Raad van State)

The Council of State is the highest legislative advisory body to the government in the Netherlands. Its members are appointed by Her Majesty the Queen. The Council's advice must be given on every bill. During the process of law making, the Second Chamber may ask for the advice of the Council of State. The advice is very important but not binding. In the area of HIVST and GDST, the Council of State has given advice on the following draft laws:

— bill regarding population sreening;

— bill regarding the medical contract;

— bill regarding additional legislation on penal sanctions against DNA investigations;

— bill regarding the handling of human embryos and gametes.

The Health Council (Gezondheidsraad)

The Health Council is a major advisor to the government. Its task, as defined in 1956 by law, is to inform the government — that is the Ministry of Health — about "the state of science relevant to issues of public health". Ethical and legal aspects are given great weight. On HIVST and GDST, advice has been given by ad hoc committees, by the Permanent Committee on AIDS, and by the Working Group on Health Ethics and Law. In return, the Council is usually informed about actions taken by the minister on the basis of its reports and advice.

The following reports concern HIVST and GDST:

— Screening for congenital metabolic diseases (1979);
— Genetic Counselling (1980);
— AIDS Problems in The Netherlands. Guidelines for group screening and advice for prevention (1986);
— AIDS: measures to protect hospital staff (1988);
— Neural tube defects (1988);
— Investigating the spread of HIV-infection in the Netherlands (1989);
— Heredity: science and society. On the potential and the limits of genetic diagnosis and gene therapy (1989);
— Early medical intervention in HIV positive persons (1990);
— Annual Advice on health care (1990);
— The HIV test and life insurance (1991);
— Medical examination and prediction. An evaluation of "An exploration of prediction in medical examination", a report by the National Institute for Public Health and Environmental Hygiene (1993).

Currently (Autumn of 1993) an opinion is being prepared on the conditions for genetic screening.

The National Commission for the campaign against AIDS

Established at the initiative of the Ministry of Health, the National Commission for the fight against AIDS (Nationale Commissie AIDS-Bestrijding) is the successor of a previous national commission for the coordination of AIDS work. This Committee offers advice, either on request or of its own initiative, to the Secretary of Health on many aspects of HIV/AIDS. The Commission's advice has a major impact upon policy. In the area of HIV testing, the following reports have been issued:

— Advice on AIDS and insurance (1987);
— Opinion on testing for antibodies against HIV (1988);
— Advice on large-scale anonymous HIV-seroprevalence investigation (1989);
— Notice on children, HIV infection and AIDS (1989);
— AIDS and personal insurance (1989);
— Financial arrangements concerning AIDS and personal insurance (1990);
— "Offside": The problems of access to insurance for those at risk of HIV infection and AIDS (1990);
— Women and AIDS (1991).

Steering Committee on Future Health Scenarios (Stuurgroep Toekomstscenario's Gezondheidszorg)

This group was established in 1983 by the Ministry of Welfare, Public Health and Culture. Its task is to develop scenario as an aid to long term health policy. For our topic, the following reports are relevant:

— Anticipating and assessing health care technology. Vol. 5: *Developments in Human Genetic Testing* (1988);

— AIDS in the Netherlands until 2000 (1992).

Recently a project called "Future scenarios on reproduction" was launched. In it, attention will be given to the ethics of biomedical technologies in the area of reproduction.

The Committee for Ethics in Medical Research (Kerncommissie Ethiek Medisch Onderzoek)

The Committee for ethics in medical research (KEMO) is a national advisory committee for the evaluation of medical and scientific research with particular ethical, legal and social content. It provides direct central support to local medical research ethics committees. Its central role attracts wide attention, including that of politicians. The advice, though not binding on local committees, has great weight. We mention the following reports:

— Annual Reports for 1989 and 1990 (1991) with a provisional opinion on the development of pre-implantation diagnosis;

— Advice on a research protocol about serum screening for women with increased risk of Down's syndrome and of neural tube defects (1992).

The Netherlands Scientific Council for Government Policy (Wetenschappelijke Raad voor het Regeringsbeleid)

The Netherlands Council for Government (WRR) does not have a section on the study of screening. It was, nevertheless, involved in 1987 in the Ministry of Health's preparation for the debate on genetics which was reported in "The social consequences of genetic testing" (1990).

The National Institute for Public Health and Environmental Hygiene (Rijksinstituut voor Volksgezondheid en Milieuhygiëne)

During 1993, this Institute published a report called "Exploration of medical prediction in medical examination"; it examined the epidemiological implications of such procedures before access to insurance and to the job market, and provided the scientific information necessary for the political and ethical debate.

The National Council for Public Health (Nationale Raad voor de Volksgezondheid)

In mid 1993, the National Council for Public Health received a request for advice from the Ministry of Health on the area of prevention. Both screening and testing will receive adequate attention in this project, which is still under way.

The National Commission for the Chronically Ill (Nationale Commissie Chronisch Zieken)

In 1991, the Secretary of Public Health installed a national commission for chronic diseases. Against the background of increasing possibilities for prenatal diagnosis, this commission will report on the conditions that ought to be met by the provision of genetic counselling.

The Netherlands Organization for Technology Assesment (Nederlandse Organisatie voor Technologisch Aspectenonderzoek)

In 1993, the Netherlands Organization for Technology Assessment (NOTA) received the minister's approval for organizing a public debate on ethical aspects of science and technology. It is likely that screening will be included. The outcome of the debates will be reported to politicians so they may integrate it in their decision making. In the near future a "Special NOTA Bulletin" will be published about sister organizations in other countries and their involvement in the Human Genome Project.

The Penal Law Reform Commission

In 1989, this Commission was asked by the Minister of Justice whether DNA fingerprinting was justified in a criminal context. In its report of January 1991, the Commission concluded that only the comparison of two samples could be justified.

The library and documentation service of the Second Chamber

The information section of the Second Chamber has three sections: Parliamentary documentation, press and periodicals, and the library.

The parliamentary documentation section contains both Dutch and official EC documents. Staff will answer all questions submitted about those sources. For the period between 1989 and 1993, apart from numerous parliamentary papers, there were four other reports on screening for HIV and three on screening for genetic disease.

The press and periodicals section surveys some 700 national and international papers and journals. A print-out of September 1993 showed the presence of 165 Dutch newspaper articles on HIV and genetic screening over the period 1989-1993, and of 60 radio and TV interviews during the same period. In all, there were 86 items on HIV and 89 on genetic. The section also draws on external data collections, both in the Netherlands and abroad (*e.g. Dialog* which is the Database on legal literature).

The third section is the Library proper. It contains books, reports, legislation, jurisprudence, statistics and parliamentary papers from foreign parliaments (Belgium, France, Germany, Luxemburg, the United Kingdom, and the USA). The greater part is legal literature. Due to current interest in issues of HIV/AIDS and genetics, the legal aspects of both have special attention. Access to "Data Juridica" — a Dutch bibliography on judicial literature — is online. The ethical literature seems less represented. No database (*e.g.* Medline, Bioethicsline) is available in the Library itself. Nevertheless, a print-out of September 1993 showed, on HIV testing, a total of forty six documents and, on genetic testing, a total of fifty one documents available within the library.

In principle, there is no limit to the search the Library and the Documentation services make: they have access to other libraries and data bases of national departments (Ministries), universities, and national institutes, as well as to a network of correspondents linking all foreign parliaments.

Experts and advisors

Both Houses of Parliament in the Netherlands have numerous permanent commissions. The relevant ones are the permanent commission of public health and the permanent commission of justice. A permanent commission has a small staff. The staff's job with incoming information is procedural, not substantive. Both the Commission and the individual Members of Parliament may invite experts and advisors. As a rule, though, the permanent commissions receive information from the coordinating minister in the government. In the case of AIDS for instance, the commission receives its information from the secretary of public health. Subsequently, it is the permanent commissions which decide the course this information will follow. Thus, the National Commission for the campaign against AIDS reports twice every year on HIV infection.

Politicians and the public

We explored two questions:

1. To what extent are politicians involved in public information about HIV and genetic screening, either as initiators or as providers of financial support?

2. Does government initiate or pay for research on what do the Dutch people think about the normative issues which arise?

Public information

We distinguish public information in the context of prevention (*e.g.* safe sex campaigns) from public information which combines scientific information with information on social and ethical aspects. Obviously, the latter, being more integral, is of greater importance to our investigation.

1. Prevention campaigns : Prevention campaigns are primarily subsidized by the Ministry of Health. Amongst the major foundations which help are the following:

— The Schorer Foundation provides public information about HIV and AIDS, *e.g.* through its AIDS-info-bulletin.

— The National Commission for the campaign against AIDS, together with the Ministry of Health, and The Foundation for Sexually Transmissible Diseases, and the AIDS Foundation, as well as the State information services form a "Project group for the public campaign against AIDS and sexually transmissible diseases". This group has a renewed campaign on safe sex. The National Commission also provides the Ministry of Health every year with an "Action plan for information on and prevention of" AIDS.

2. Integral information : The word "integral" means here scientific, social, and ethical information on either HIV/AIDS or Genetics. The following organizations are involved:

— The Foundation for Public Information on Science and Technology (PWT), subsidized by the Ministries of Education/Science and of Economic Affairs, edits information files on AIDS and on prenatal diagnosis. These are available on demand. For 1994, a project on "Medical Biotechnology" is programmed. Genetic diagnosis will be included, and the product will be a brochure and a TV programme on genetic testing.

— The Biosciences and Society Foundation publishes "Notes" in both fields. Thus, 2 Notes on AIDS, 1 on DNAdiagnostics, and 1 on pre-embryo research. Subsidies come from the Ministries of Education/Science and of Economic Affairs.

— The Association of Collaborating Organizations of Parents and Patients (VSOP) illustrates the mix of science and social/ethical aspects in the field of genetics. Information in view of prevention is combined with information on the state of the art and progress in science, as well as on social and ethical aspects. With the support of the ministry of health, a national ethics project on Heredity resulted in an "Ethical Manifesto" *(see below)* and a national convention "Choice not Chance". A manual on "Ethics and heredity" was also developed.

Government supported opinion polls

We were not able to find any trace of such things.

Other bodies and their reports

Political parties and their study bureaux

Of the many political parties in The Netherlands it is commonly agreed that four have the highest profiles. They are, the Christian Democrats (CDA), the Socialists (PvdA), the Liberals (VVD), and Democracy '66 (D66).

The Christian Democrats' Scientific Institute published a report on "Genes and limits; a Christian Democratic contribution to the debate on gene technology" (1992). The following recommendations were made:

— government ought to lay down criteria for establishing centres of Clinical Genetics. Indeed it is the government's duty to counter possible tendencies in medicalization and in medicine which merely fulfill people's wishes;
— prenatal screening with abortion as the only possible outcome ought to be legally prohibited;
— preimplantation diagnosis by embryo splitting should be prohibited;
— specific hereditary testing as a condition for additional insurance ought to be rejected;
— genetic testing as a condition to obtain a job ought to be forbidden;
— DNA testing against the suspect's will should be admitted only for serious crimes and under strict conditions.

The Socialist Party's Working Group on Biotechnology published a report "To live and let live" (1993), in which the following recommendations were made:

— no prior conditions ought to be set to genetic investigation;

— genetic investigation ought to occur only in the best interest of the individual and his/her offspring;
— genetic tests in the context of insurance or job applications ought to be forbidden. It is logical that no further questions be asked about the incidence of hereditary diseases in the family;
— genetic screening may occur only under the strictest conditions;
— regarding preimplantation diagnosis a 'no, unless' policy is indicated.

The Liberals' Telders Foundation is currently preparing a report on genetics.

Democracy '66 has a Scientific Bureau. Its periodical *IDEE* will, in the near future, publish a series of articles on our subjects of HIVST and GDST without, however, engaging the Bureau. A Working Group "Faith and political action" finished, in the Summer of 1993, a report on prenatal diagnosis (particularly on preimplantation diagnosis) and on germline gene therapy. It still has to be decided whether the report can be published as an official document of the Bureau.

Churches and non-denominational groups

1. The Churches

The Roman Catholic Church works through the researchservices of the catholic bishops' conference (BK). BK organizes yearly one or two contacts with two major political parties (Christian Democrats and Socialists) on issues of public health and ethics. In 1987 an episcopal declaration on AIDS was issued. In this document the bishops expressed particular concern for AIDS patients and seropositive individuals. They also warn against the danger of discrimination. Their declaration says nothing about HIV screening. Nor has genetic screening yet been on the agenda of the catholic research services. The current interest for organ transplantation, in view of a recent draft law on the matter, may lead to the inclusion of a passage on screening for genetic disorders.

The Netherlands Reformed Church (Hervormde Kerk) communicates with Parliament through its Council on government and society, which, in turn, is usually briefed by a committee on Church and health care. While both areas of screening have the attention of the Committee, no position on either area has yet been taken. In 1987 a pastoral letter on AIDS was issued. Its content was very similar to that of the letter issued by the Roman Catholic Church: the need for pastoral care and human support amongst seropositive individuals and AIDS patients.

The Reformed Churches of the Netherlands *(Gereformeerde Kerken)* do not often contact MPs, and have no plans to do so in this field.

The Multidisciplinary Centre for Church and Society informs parliament and various ministries on the issues of biotechnology and ethics. In 1989 this Centre launched a petition to the Houses of Representatives demanding that, of all money voted for the development of technolgy, 4% be put aside for ethical debate. No immediate reaction was registered, but, in 1992, the Ministry of Education and Science showed renewed interest in the matter. This lead to a report on "codes of ethics and the social responsibility of technologists". Genetics has not been on the agenda since 1988, but there will shortly be attention to it. AIDS has not been on the agenda.

2. The Association of Humanists *(Humanistisch Verbond)*

An *ad hoc* committee formed by members of both the Netherlands and the Flanders associations published in 1990 "Biosociety: a humanistic view on the ethics of biomedicine". The following recommendations amongst others were made:

— prenatal diagnosis ought to be used only in the fight against pathological deviations;
— in medical examinations and tests, the principles of privacy and informed consent ought to be respected.

Some incidental statements have also been issued by the Association:

— one was issued after press reports about involuntary HIV testing of patients before operations. Support for informed consent was reaffirmed, and the authorities were asked to condemn such practices (March 1988);

— in April 1989, the proposal made by the Health Council for wide screening for HIV without informed consent brought a second statement of rejection from the Board of the Association.

All these viewpoints were made known to Parliament. The Association's view is put by its President, who is a Member of the Senate.

Research Institutes and Universities

1. **Government**: Under its research programme "Ethics and law", the Ministry of Welfare, Public Health and Culture (WVC) has contracted out a number of projects on HIVST and GDST to the Institute for Social Medicine (Amsterdam), to the Center for Bioethics and Health Law (Utrecht) and to the Institute for Bioethics (Maastricht):

— Institute for Social Medicine (University of Amsterdam):

- Medical examination and employment (1990);
- Genetic information, employment, and employment related benefits (1993-1995).

— Institute for Bioethics and Health Law (University of Utrecht):

- Aids and ethics (1989);
- HIV infection, insurances and jobs (1990);
- HIV infection and access to health care (1991).

Institute for Bioethics (Maastricht):

- Ethics and screening for carriers of genetic defects (1989);

- Genetic information and life insurance: ethical and legal aspects (1991);
- Predictive genetic testing (1993-1995).

2. Universities and other centres for ethics and health law have initiated the following research on HIVST and GDST:

— The Department of Health Law, University of Limburg:

- Drug research against HIV infection (1990);
- Criminal and civil liability (1990);
- Testing for HIV antibodies (1990);
- International migration and HIV infection (1991);
- Risk selection by private insurers within the CEC (1991);
- Health care and the risk of HIV infection (1991);
- Access to health care (1991).

— The department of the history of medicine, Catholic University Nijmegen: The human genome and body identity (a CEC research project).

— The department of medical ethics, University Leiden: Ethical dilemmas of clinical genetics.

— Institute for ethics, Free University of Amsterdam: Ethics and presymptomatic diagnosis of late onset disease.

— The Pr. Dr. G.A. Lindeboom Institute (Ede):
- Prenatal diagnosis: policy towards indications and cover by health care insurance (1989);
- HIV testing versus genetic testing (1989);
- HIV testing: compulsory or not? (1989).

All these reports, as well as occasional letters, were sent to the members of Parliament and/or ministers.

— The Netherlands Institute of Human Rights (in collaboration with the Danish Centre for Human Rights): AIDS and human rights in the European communities (1992).

Medical and scientific organizations

1. The Association for Health Law *(Vereniging voor Gezondheidsrecht)*. This association has twice advised the government about screening for HIV and genetic disease:

— A position paper on testing for antibodies against HIV at the moment of application for insurance (1988). This paper comments on the Minister of Justice's white paper to the Second Chamber on the legal aspects of insurance for people at risk of AIDS. The paper pleads for better protection of individuals under medical examination.

— Guidelines on hereditary investigation (1991). The report recommends legislation on the following points:

• informing clients on the (possible) use of genetic information and body material for other purposes than individual health services;
• the client's right to allow or to forbid registration of genetic information and the preservation of body material for other purposes than health services to the client;
• protection of the candidate in applications for insurance and employment against any invitation to collaborate with genetic investigation.

2. The Dutch Royal Medical Association *(Koninklijke Nederlandse Maatschappij tot Bevordering der Geneeskunst)*.

This association has repeatedly expressed its views on HIV and genetic screening.

— A position paper on HIV testing in medical examination (1990). HIV testing on principle ought not to be done in medical examinations. An exception to the rule would be an examination for an individual life insurance of more than 200,000 Florins. Also, should there be obvious medical indications of seropositivity, and according to the importance of diagnosis for the individual examinee, HIV-testing should be permitted. Several conditions, *e.g.* informed consent, must be respected.

— A position paper on blood sampling for DNA-investigation of (criminally) suspected persons (1991), asked for by the Ministry of Justice. Should legislation on this be introduced, there seems to be no medical ethical objection against a physician's participation in blood taking, provided a few conditions are met: *e.g.*, crimes that justify DNA-investigation ought to be listed in the Criminal Code.

3. Dutch Association for Obstetrics and Gynaecology *(Nederlandse Vereniging voor Obstetrie en Gynecologie).* This Association has issued two important reports:

— "Prenatal Diagnosis" (1992). This report draws the following conclusions:

• parental autonomy ought to be the basic principle guiding government;
• prenatal diagnosis of untreatable late-onset diseases is irresponsible unless abortion is being considered;
• extreme restraint is required when genetic information may be used by employers and insurance companies.

— Report "Late abortion" (1992). A late abortion, performed during the third trimester, is illegal in the Netherlands. Nevertheless, in cases of very serious fetal defects, the question of late abortion arises. This report offers guidelines for the gynaecologist.

4. Dutch Association for Clinical Genetics *(Vereniging Klinische Genetica Nederland).* This association has a constant interest in ethical issues. However, its opinions are not public.

Interest groups

1. Insurance companies. Currently the Union of Insurers of the Netherlands is gathering several existing insurers' organizations into a single Union. This regrouping is relevant to this report, because one single voice may result in one clear and loud message.

How do insurers inform the members of Parliament? Whenever useful or necessary, *e.g.* when new bills are being tabled, or when positions of politicians or interest groups reach Parliament, the Dutch insurers will speak up. First, they systematically address in writing the pertinent Committees and only those: for instance the Finance, Public Health, and Justice Committees. Second, the insurers have personal meetings with the leaders of political parties. Third, they lobby amongst politicians: this lobbying includes a final update immediately before the debate in the Second Chamber. The insurers also seem to carefully follow and critically scrutinize ethical end legal reports in the field. Critiques and comments are sent to the members of Parliament.

The insurers have also developed intense contacts with various Ministries. Policy makers and legal advisors are well informed of the views of the insurers. The latter agreed with the ministers of health, finance, and justice in 1989 that applicants should not be asked to undergo HIV testing, and that insurance below 200,000 Florins should be free of the obligation to offer information on HIV/AIDS. An identical voluntary agreement was reached on genetic testing and information in 1990.

2. Main patient organizations

— The Association of Collaborating Parents and Patients Organizations (Vereniging van Samenwerkende Ouder- en Patintenorganisaties). In 1990, this Association published its "Ethical Manifesto", partly as a reaction against the Notice "Congenital defects". Normative principles and recommendations for policy are stated in order to stimulate debate amongst government and relevant institutions. During the national congress on "Choice not chance" (1990) the manifesto was handed to the Secretary of Health. It was also sent to the members of Parliament. It states that government ought to secure that:

- distribution of information on genetic investigation and education be stimulated;

- the genetic constitution of people does not interfere with their living, work, and insurance arrangements;
- genetic examinations should never be imposed;
- all possibilities should be used to stimulate a climate of social solidarity towards those with a handicap and towards their families.

— Broad Insurance Platform (*Breed Platform Verzekeringen:* BPV). This is an umbrella organization of thirteen patient and consumer organizations. Its aim is to reinforce the legal position of applicants for insurance. The Platform claims that a person's present medical status ought to be the standard for the issuing of a policy. This means that it is not acceptable for an insurer to ask either for already known predictive information or for additional predictive testing for genetic disorders or HIV. This viewpoint has been repeatedly made known to MPs.

— The Dutch Association of Haemophilia Patients. Through frequent contacts with government and with insurers this association tries to protect the interests of its members. Insurers deemed it justified to test all haemophilia applicants (even below 200,000 Florins) for HIV, because of the extra risk. This would have been an exception to the voluntary agreement. It was decided instead to set up an insurance guarantee fund with money from the government. This made the request for HIV-testing of Haemophiliac appplicants (for an insurance below 200,000 Florins) superfluous.

— The Dutch HIV Association. This interest group has addressed Parliament several times with policy recommendations. For instance, it stated that insurers, in the context of the so-called "health declaration" are, in the Association's view, entitled to ask applicants for insurance only whether they have AIDS, and not whether they are seropositive. They claimed that healthy, asymptomatic HIV infected individuals must not be excluded from insurance, meaning life insurance as well (1992).

3. Others : The Dutch association for the integration of homosexuality (Nederlandse Vereniging voor de integratie van Homosexualiteit). This association has told the government that they opposed HIV testing of applicants for insurance. Regarding the recent debate on the "homo-gene", the COC has published its opinion in the major daily papers saying that the social appropriateness of such testing was doubtful and that, in their circle, there was no interest in obtaining further knowledge in the area.

Survey of Parliamentary debates, issues and legislation

Survey of debates in Parliament

(All references refer to the official Publications of the Second Chamber *Tweede Kamerstukken*; except for the references where other sources, *e.g.* the First Chamber, are mentioned).

1. Debate on the white paper on prevention of congenital defects (1987-1989, 20 345, nrs. 1-5);

2. Debate on population screening for neural tube defects (occasioned by a position taken by the Ministry of Health after the Health Council's advice on NTD) (1989-1992, 21 353, nrs. 1-3);

3. Debate on draft law about Population screening (1988-1992, 21 264; nrs. 1-20) (First Chamber 1991-1992, 21 264, nr. 283, 283A, 283B) (Acts II 1991-1992, pp. 3746-3768; 3799-3824; 4406-4408; 4623-4624) (Acts I, 1992-1993, nr. 004, p. 161);

4. Debate on genetic diagnosis and gene therapy (occasioned by the joint letter of the Minister of Justice and the Secretary of Health (November 30th, 1990) regarding the Health Council's advisory report "Heredity: science and society") (1990-1992, 21 948. nrs. 1-7) (Acts II 1991-1992);

5. Debate on white paper on AIDS (1985-1986, 19 218, nrs. 1-4);

6. Report of deliberation by the permanent commission for public health on the Health Council's opinion on reporting of AIDS (1985-1986, 19 218, nr. 5);

7. Debate on the white paper regarding AIDS policy (1986-1987, 19 218, nr. 9; and 1987-1988, 19218, nrs 11, 12, 13);

8. White paper regarding juridical aspects of insurance in situations of AIDS-risk (1987-1988, 19 218, nrs. 10, 27, 28; and 1988-1989, 19 218, nr. 29);

9. Debate concerning the white paper on AIDS and medical examination of job applicants, and the white paper on aspects of applicants' and workers' rights when they are seropositive (1987-1988; 19 218, nrs. 15, 16, 18, 21; and 1989-1990, 19 218, nrs. 32, 33, 37, 40; and 1990-1991, 19 218, nr. 45);

10. Debate on reports of the Health Council "Investigation and spread of HIV-infection in the Netherlands", and the National Commission for the campaign against AIDS "Anonymous large scale seroprevalence screening" (1989-1990, 19 218, nrs. 39, 43; and 1991-1992, 19 218, nr. 52), and the draft law on the medical contract (WGBO): 1991-1992, 21 561, nr. 11, p. 17 where large-scale prevalence screening on the basis of an opting out system is mentioned);

11. Debate on the white paper on AIDS/seropositivity, genetic investigation and insurance (1989-1990, 19 218, nrs. 41, 43; and 1990-1991, 19 218, nr. 47; and 1991-1992, 19 218, nrs. 49, 51, 54);

12. Progress report on AIDS policy (1991-1992, 19 218, nr. 48);

13. Debate on HIV testing during pregnancy (1985-1986, 19 218, nr. 5, p. 9; 1986-1987, 19 218, nrs. 8-9, p. 21-23, 1991-1992, 19 218, nr. 48, p. 36);

14. Debate on forensic DNA research (Draft law, number 22 447; Advice State Council, 1991-1992, 22 447, A + B; 1992-1993, 22 447, nr. 6, p. 9).

Main issues debated in Parliament

It is useful to distinguish two areas where testing and screening may be applied, in health care and outside it. In surveying issues debated in Parliament we shall follow that division.

1. Within health care

— *Genetic counselling*

• The aim of genetic counselling: Both parliament and government agree that the primary goal of counselling is to meet the need of clients for adequate information to enable them to make a well informed choice of their own. The opinion that government would be entitled to push genetic counselling as an instrument of population eugenics for the sake of lower morbidity and mortality, is rejected by parliament and government alike. Nor is prenatal diagnosis seen as a "search and destroy mission", but rather as a means to inform clients who will decide by themselves to carry on with a pregnancy or not.

• The legal position of those who seek counselling: Great importance is attached to the client's right to be informed, his right not to know if he refuses information, and his right to privacy for his genetic information. The latter two rights are perceived as being important but not absolute. Serious injury to relatives may override the client's right in a conflict of duties.

— *Prenatal diagnosis*

• Indications for prenatal diagnosis : As possibilities for diagnosing ever more (also less serious) defects increase, so the discussion about indications for prenatal diagnosis continues. A debate about meaningful medical indications is necessary. The use and abuse of prenatal chromosomal diagnosis for sex selection determined by social criteria, as well as the age limit (36 years in the Netherlands) for chromosomal prenatal diagnosis, are issues under debate. Concerning the latter, the question of lowering the age limit has been raised.

- Declaration of intent: Given a valid medical indication for prenatal diagnosis, access should not be limited to patients who express their willingness to have an abortion if the fetus is affected. Such policy might prove to be coercive prevention. But untreatable late onset diseases make poignant cases. Indeed, when after a positive test result, the pregnancy is not terminated, this might mean the child would be heavily burdened by the knowledge.

- Preimplantation diagnosis: This latest technology raises several controversial issues. First, it is questionable whether this form of diagnosis is justified and desirable. Second, it raises the issue of non-therapeutic experiments on human embryos, a necessary phase before the technology can be safely introduced in the clinic. Parliament might attach great importance to the possible difference between experimenting on left over embryos and creating embryos for the sole purpose of research. Recently a draft law was tabled in the Second Chamber.

— *Genetic screening*

- The duty to report intended screening programmes: There is unanimity on the desirability of restricting population screening through a system of licensing. The consensus is based on the need to protect the population against potential dangers for physical or mental health. The precise content of such regulation is debated. There is a difference of opinion regarding the advantages and disadvantages of a general duty to report intended genetic screening in advance. Thus, for the sake of the highest possible security, some want to be certain that intended population screening programmes will be permanently surveyed, thus allowing intervention where necessary. Others deny that such a general duty to report would offer any new value to the information already available in the Health Council's report on (intended) screening programmes.

- Postnatal screening for serious diseases or abnormalities for which no treatment or prevention is available: There is a consensus that such screening should require permission. Some argue that permission should always be refused, others would allow it for a few exceptional cases.

• Prenatal population screening: Maternal Serum Alpha-Foeto-Protein (MSAFP) screening is a most controversial issue. By means of such biochemical screening during pregnancy, one could identify women with an increased risk of having a child with a neural tube defect or with some chromosomal disorder. It is crucial to know whether such screening meets the general screening criteria. The widely held requirement that one screens only within a context of accepted therapy does not apply, since termination of pregnancy could be the only possible outcome. Parliament is unanimous in calling this neither prevention nor treatment. Some see the need for total prohibition, others for general refusal of permission, leaving room only for a rare exceptional case.

• Carrier screening: Screening people in order to identify those individuals who carry recessive hereditary diseases is generally considered to fall within the scope of licensing. There is a difference of opinion, however, about the rightness of licensing it. For some people, the enormous psychic burden for carriers is a sufficient reason to refuse licensing. Others deem such a refusal premature and wish to weigh various aspects more carefully. They are convinced that the possibility of being informed about genetic risk, prior to a pregnancy, is, in principle, useful.

— *HIV testing*

HIV testing of patients is permitted only on medical indication and provided he/she has given informed consent. As a contagious disease AIDS/HIV must be reported to the inspection of Public Health. However, the precarious character of the disease causes it to be limited to free and anonymous reporting. The government also deems that a physician is not obliged to inform the partner of a seropositive patient. The matter is left to the physician's judgment.

In Parliament, special attention has been paid to routine HIV testing of pregnant women and to compulsory testing of prostitutes addicted to heroin, but the government did not accept either proposal. In pregnant women, the seroprevalence is so low that the financial cost outweighs routine testing, and heroin prostitutes are put under extra health surveillance.

As for large scale, HIV prevalence screening of the Dutch population, the government felt that such screening was not justified because of the lack of a national health interest.

In HIV testing, both government and parliament emphasize information and prevention. National information campaigns are meant to influence the general public and particular groups. Those to be tested should be fully informed about the advantages and disadvantages of the test, and about their right not to know. It is the government's view that both information and consent are sufficiently regulated in the draft law on the Medical Contract.

2. Outside health care

— Labour and insurance

It seems that the outcome of the debates on AIDS and HIV testing has set the trend for coping with the problems of genetic testing. In medical examinations for both jobs and insurance, the HIV test regulations have often influenced the way genetic testing is handled.

The basic problem underlying HIV and genetic testing for insurance and job applications is twofold. First, in the Netherlands, job application generally implies that one may be submitted to medical examination to determine one's suitability for the job and for the company's pension scheme. Secondly, different kinds of insurance policies serve different purposes. Thus, for instance, medical examinations for life and health insurance may be more thorough than they are for pensions. Therefore difficulties may arise in setting out a general policy on both

HIV and genetic testing. Yet, to cope with the diversity in testing policies, steps are taken to come to a uniform set of medical criteria, by means of consultation among the secretary of State for health care, the royal Dutch medical association and the Medical advisors of the insurers).

In general, the government strongly recommends restraint in testing and screening. Here are some specific examples:

• HIV, job application and pension scheme. The government has stated that medical examination for job application and pension scheme is to be restricted solely to the determination of suitability for the job. From the standpoint of industrial law, no discrimination is allowed between HIV positive and other applicants. If asked, the applicant may rightly refuse to answer questions about his or her HIV serostatus. Furthermore, the government is of the opinion that neither HIV positivity nor AIDS should be ground for dismissal. Should the applicant suffer from AIDS, the government thinks it reasonable that the applicant, if asked, should inform the employer.

• HIV and job application in the army. Medical examination, including HIV testing in the military is excluded. This is in line with the government's view on medical examination in job application by civilians. In this case the law on military medical examination is applicable. In special circumstances, although under strong protest, HIV testing was accepted (*e.g.* participants in the Security Assistance Training Programm (SATP)).

• Job application and genetic information. The Government has decreed that, in the job application context, no examination of hereditary predisposition must take place. As to the use of genetic testing so as to be able to prevent occupational diseases, the government told parliament that current possibilities were quite limited, but that they will most attentively follow further developments. Parliament seems to be unanimous in saying that such medical examinations may only address what is directly relevant to medical fitness for the job concerned. With regard to the possible use of genetic screening and testing to prevent occupational diseases, parliament is of the opinion that a well applied law on working conditions is to be preferred. Industry should never be allowed to screen in order to determine which labourer should go to what unhealthy spot in the plant. Parliament has voted in favour of the introduction of a law excluding genetic screening and testing related to occupational disease.

• Different kinds of insurance policies. The issues of HIV and genetic testing are felt most strongly in two kinds of insurances: (private) industrial disability policies, and life policies. Medical examination for these kinds of policy aims at the evaluation of health risks. Therefore, in general, the government feels it reasonable that the insurer should try to identify these risks, which are own. Because of the major problems for the individual, such as stigmatization or discrimination as well as psychological problems, and the fact that no consensus has yet been reached, government and insurance companies made a voluntary agreement that: (1) there will be no active use of genetic screening or testing; (2) for a five year period (starting 1990), applicants for life insurance are not obliged to report genetic information they already possess, nor can they be submitted to an HIV test, as long as the total amount of the life insurance does not exceed 200,000 florins (that is approximately 93,000 ECUS) and the amount of the industrial disability insurance does not exceed 60,000 florins, that is approximately 28,000 ECUS, in the first year and 40,000 florins, that is approximately 19,000 ECUS, in the second year. This voluntary agreement will be evaluated when the five year term is over, that is during 1994. Meanwhile, it must be said that parliament is not satisfied with it. Parliament has passed a motion asking the government to provide legislation on the matter. It would seem that the government's delay has led to the recently tabled draft law 23 259.

It is being suggested that the government should arrange a special kind of financial pool on behalf of HIV seropositive people in order to make it easier for them to get insurance. However the government is of the opinion that such a pool will not solve these problems (testing will still be necessary). Besides, pooling wold constitutes a discrimination against other patient groups.

— *Forensic DNA*

Some years ago, the Minister of Justice asked the Penal Law Reform Commission to investigate the feasibility of DNA profile sampling of suspects of serious criminal offences. *(See also above.)* The commission concluded that under strict regulations (in view of the constitution and of treaties on human rights) the use of DNA technology was justified. No genetic information is gathered, nor is it possible to use the suspect's material for any other kind of test, like HIV. The conclusion of the commission is in a draft law (number 22 447) and awaits approval of the First Chamber.

Accepted draft laws

The Bill on Genetic Screening was accepted in 1992. Meanwhile, however, its introduction is awaiting a General Ordinance of Order.

Draft laws on HIV and genetic testing

1. Bill on the handling of human embryos and gametes. This draft law is relevant to preimplantation diagnosis. It allows the minister to call for a moratorium on experiments with human embryos, should self regulation by the professions prove to be insufficient. Such a moratorium would impede, for the time being, preclinical research on human embryos in order to develop a preimplantation diagnosis. The draft law prohibits the creation of embryos for scientific research. The draft law considers totipotent blastomeres to be embryos, meaning that they would also be excluded. There are rumours that the Minister is about to submit a revised draft law for advice to the Council of State.

2. Draft law on medical examinations of applicants. The draft law (tabled by D 66) intends to reinforce the position of the applicant for life, pension and (private) disability insurance policies. Only general rules are formulated. The implementation is left to self-regulation by insurers, employers, consumers and physicians. The core statement of the draft law is that questions and medical examinations must all relate to the purposes of the examination. Means and ends should be reasonably related to each other. In order to monitor developments, an independent commission to receive complaints should be established.

3. The draft law on forensic DNA comparisons (nr. 22 447). This draft law proposes that such DNA comparisons be only acceptable for serious crimes, *i.e.* crimes that could be punished with more than eight years of imprisonment.

4. Draft law on the Medical Contract (WGBO). This draft law intends to secure certain patient's rights, *e.g.* the right to be informed or not to be informed and the right to look into one's medical record. It also stipulates that informed consent must be obtained prior to every medical act. In the light of this draft law, HIVST and GDST would only be possible after informed consent has been obtained. A special section of the draft law sees to "leftovers" of human material and stipulates that in, medical research, an opting out system concerning these materials might be possible, provided that the anonymity of the subjects is guaranteed.

The well informed MP

We interviewed five members of the Second Chamber. They were: Mrs. M. Janmaat-Abee (Christian Democrat, spokeswoman on HIV and genetic screening and testing), Mr. J. Kohnstamm (Democracy '66), Mrs. F.J. Laning-Boersema (Christian Democrat, spokeswoman on genetic screening and testing), Mrs. T. Netelenbos (Socialist), and Mrs. E.G. Terpstra (Liberal). All seemed generally satisfied with the delivery times of reports and material. While Parliamentarians rarely find time to read all scientific information themselves, they do regret that universities and research institutes all too often forget to translate research into social and policy recommendations. All our interviewees are also members of the permanent committee of the Second Chamber on public health and health care. Their need is for information which is scientifically sound, yet translated into its social and policy implications. Furthermore, they seemed to think that a keen personal interest in the subject matter is essential if one is going to be well informed. It is, therefore, a question of activating the flow of fact-finding and information about society.

Generally, the flow of information seems to be generated by the major parties and those other parties that form with them the coalition government. They set the agenda for debate. Moreover, they also have foreknowledge of topics to come and may find time to prepare themselves. Sometimes, they get interim results from special committees. Then, they can stimulate ministries to contract out studies and receive relevant information directly and early. In other words, major parties inform themselves "proactively". Minor parties, or at least the parties which do not participate in government, on the other hand, inform themselves "retroactively". They tend to feel as if they are constantly overtaken by events.

A common remark made by our MPs was that in the Netherlands, chronologically speaking, the "HIV issues" came to the attention of the politicians first and therefore set a frame within which, subsequently, some genetic issues were also handled. Thus AIDS has been perceived by many politicians as a test bed for genetic screening and testing.

Another point all of our interviewees agreed on was that personal and bilateral contacts are a prime source for information. Contacts with care providers, patients, patient organizations and other interest groups will gradually spin a web of information. This multiplicity of informants seems to be essential to obtain quality information about the society as a whole and all the social aspects of a given problem such as HIV and Genetic Disease.

While we had the impression that both major and minor party spokespersons were quite well informed, they themselves admitted that the average MP who is not a member of the permanent commission on public health and health care is not as well informed as the party's spokesperson in the field.

Bioethics in the Portuguese Parliament

ALBERTO MARTINS[1], JOSÉ LEITAO[2]

The debating of issues related to bioethics or, in a broader sense, to the life sciences, is fairly recent in the Portuguese Parliament and so far has dealt with a limited range of questions.

In 1986, Mr Mário Raposo, the then Minister of Justice, created a Committee for legislating on New Technologies which would work within the Ministry of Justice, but most of the work done by that Committee had no follow-up. The first draft of the bill written at the time wasn't available until 1990, when it was published by the Center for Biomedical Law of the University of Coimbra Law School.

In 1989, the Parliamentary Group of the Socialist Party organized a parliamentary seminar in which renowned specialists in bioethics participated. This seminar led to the creation of the National Committee on Ethics for the Life Sciences (henceforth, NCELS).

The parliamentary debate which triggered interest in these matters led to the creation of the NCELS (Law no. 14/90 of June 9th, based on a bill presented by the Socialist Party and,

---

1. Member of Parliament.
2. Former member of Parliament.

later, on a bill presented by the governing Social-Democratic Party).

The fact that the press often focuses on the ethical conflicts raised by the progress of the life sciences has affected both parliamentary activity, by increasing the importance given to those matters, and the activities of the parliamentary support structures.

Information about the life sciences within Parliament

The debate about the creation of the NCELS took place in 1990, without any specialized support available to members, and before the possibility of parliamentary hearings was established by parliamentary rules. Later on, more information on issues related to the life sciences was made available to members.

The DILP — Division of Legislative and Parliamentary Information (Divisao de Informaçao Legislative e Parlamentar) — undertook studies on:

— Ethics Council — April 1992;

— Medically Assisted Fertilization (Use of embryos) — April 1992;

— Transplants and removal of Human Organs and Tissues (Number I) — April 1992;

— Transplants and removal of Human Organs and Tissues (Number II — addenda containing foreign legislative texts) — April 1992;

— Transsexuality — June 1992;

— Transsexuality (Number II — addenda containing Legislation, Jurisprudence and foreign doctrines) — June 1992;

— Voluntary Interruption of Pregnancy — July 1992.

These studies were not undertaken specifically to support parliamentary debate, although their interest is undeniable. The parliamentary library has collected four volumes of associated documentation as well as some papers on bioethical issues. These were also compiled and organized in 1992. A brief description of the contents of each of them follows:

— Volume 1: General Framework. Number 1: Introduction: general framework. Number 2: Scientific research: general framework. Addendum 1: The FAST Programme. Addendum 2: Euthanasia.

— Volume 2: Number 1: Use of the embryo and fetus: a comparative analysis. Addendum to Number 2: Medically Assisted Fertilization: the French Senate Study.

— Volume 3: Organ and tissue removal and transplants: a comparative analysis.

— The following papers on Bioethics were also published:

— Fertilization Medicine. Number 1: Germany. Number 2: United Kingdom.

— Bioethical Issues. Number 1: Portugal — European and International Organizations. Number 2: Comparative data: support texts.

— Abortion Law.

The revision of the legislation on removal of tissues for transplants resulted in an important debate.

The socialist party bill N° 40/VI and Government Bill N° 9/VI were widely debated at the Parliament's plenary session during 1992, and the committee debate resulted in a text which received a broad acceptance. The new law, N° 12/93, of April 22nd, regulates administrative procedures for the donation or removal of human tissues or organs for diagnosis, therapeutic or transplant purposes, as well as the surgical procedures themselves. It does not apply to the donation of ova and sperm, the transfer or handling of embryos, or blood transfusions; but it regulates the removal of human tissues and organs from both live and dead subjects.

Removal from minors and from disabled persons was given special attention. Donor consent to removal where the donor is living must, in the case of minors, be given by the parents, unless they are prohibited from exercising parental authority by a court of law. In this case or in the absence of both parents, consent must be given by a court. The donation of tissues or organs by fully understanding minors who are capable of informed consent, also requires the minor's agreement. Organ removal from mentally-disabled adults is permitted only by court order.

In the case of organ removal from corpses, the law considers as potential post mortem donors all Portuguese citizens, stateless persons and foreigners living in Portugal, who have not informed the Ministry of Health that they do not wish to be donors, either in respect of any organ or tissue, or in respect of particular organs or tissues, or where a particular use is to be made of the bodily donation.

A computerized National Record of Non-Donors (RENNDA) was created to record the names of the citizens who have expressed their wish not to be donors. Minors and disabled citizens may be declared non-donors, for the purpose of this record, by their legal representatives. Fully understanding minors who are capable of informed consent can also declare themselves non-donors.

Contamination by the human immunodeficiency virus (HIV), and the use of contaminated blood in transfusions, has been frequently addressed. Between October 1988 and July 1994, parliamentarians referred to it 85 times, including questions to the government. It can also be mentioned that there is a government-run National Committee for the Fight Against AIDS.

In the present legislative term (the sixth, from 1991 to 1995) two bills concerning HIV have been presented: N° 145/VI, on the prevention and treatment of infection by HIV (DAR, 2nd series — A — N° 38); and N° 146/VI, on compensation to persons infected by the HIV in the process of a blood transfusion (DAR, 2nd series — a — N° 38). The bills, presented by socialist party members, were both rejected by the Social-Democratic majority.

Medically-assisted fertilization has not yet been the subject of a parliamentary debate. It is currently practised, although on a small scale, regulated by the following limited legislation: Article No 1839 of the Civil Code, which determines that paternity cannot be contested on grounds that the woman consented to be artificially inseminated; and Article 214 of the Penal Code, which determines that an individual who artificially inseminates a woman without her consent shall be sentenced to one to five years in prison. Obviously, criminal prosecution depends on a criminal complaint being filed. Law N° 319/86, of September 25th, establishes some norms relating to the activity of sperm banks.

The lack of a specialized library

There isn't a library that specializes in bioethics in the Portuguese Parliament. However, in the last few years there has been a growing interest in the subject, due to the need to provide information for the Council. Article No 2 of Law No 14/90, which created the NCELS, states that the parliamentary library services must collaborate with the council.

Subscriptions to periodicals

The library subscribes to the following foreign periodicals: *Journal International de Bioéthique, Lettre du Comité Consultatif National d'Éthique pour les Sciences de la Vie,* and *Ethica,* edited by the French Senator Franck Sérusclat. It also receives some Portuguese publications, such as *Cadernos de Bio-*

Etica, and publications of the Center for Biomedical Law of the University of Coimbra.

Interested committees

There isn't a committee in charge of debating the issues raised by bioethics. The bills mentioned above were debated in the Parliamentary Committee for Constitutional Affairs, Rights, Freedom and Guarantees, and/or in the Parliamentary Health Committee.

Public hearings

Public hearings were not considered in the law until the last revision of parliament rules. Taking advantage of this new possibility, and by the initiative of the Portuguese Communist Party, Parliamentary Hearing N° 25/VI was held in 1994. It focused on the infection with HIV of persons who had received transfusions at public health facilities (DAR II, B Series, 30, 25/6/94). On the initiative of the Parliament's Health Committee, a Parliamentary Colloquium on "Ethical and Legal Aspects of the Use of Corpses for Teaching and Research Purposes" was held on June 28, 1994.

External information

It is not a tradition of Portuguese parliamentary history to maintain formal, institutionalized relations with pressure groups, industries, churches or lobbyists. Therefore, the only institutionalized relation is with the NCELS, which analyses the moral questions raised by scientific progress in the fields of biology, medicine and health. Although the Council is under the Office of the Prime Minister, and not under Parliament, as had been suggested in the Socialist Party's bill, it nonetheless has an institutional relation with Parliament.

The parliament appoints to the NCELS six persons whose expertise and moral character are well known, taking into account the main ethical and religious currents (Article N° 3 of Law N° 14/90).

Parliament can, on the initiative of its President, or of one twentieth of its members, request the Council's opinion. The President of the Republic, Cabinet members, and other bodies entitled to appoint members, as well as public or private facilities where procedures are used that may have ethical implications in the areas of biology, medicine or health, can also ask the Council for an opinion.

The Council was consulted about the parliament bill and the government bill on organ and tissue removal for transplants (1/CNE/91).

The Council has made recommendations on:

— the use of corpses for research and teaching purposes (2/CNE/92);

— medically assisted fertilization (3/CNE/93);

— clinical testing of drugs (4/CNE/93 and 5/CNE/93);

— criteria for determining brain death (6/CNE/94);

— on the legal protection of biotechnological inventions (7/CNE/94).

In March 1992, the council organized a seminar on "Informed Consent", at which renowned Portuguese and foreign experts were present, and which preceded the publication of legislation on this subject proposed by the government.

On March 5, 1994, the Council organized a seminar on the functioning of the Ethics Council and its relation to the NCELS. These initiatives had a significant impact and will certainly influence parliament's legislative activity.

The Portuguese parliament has been, unicameral, since the revolution of 1974. The "Assembleia da República" has 230 Deputies, representing eight political parties. Four small parties have been elected in a coalition with another party. Elections are held in electoral districts whose boundaries are established by law. The members are elected according to the system of proportional representation, Hondt's method of the highest average.

Bioethics in the Spanish Parliament

MARCELO PALACIOS[1]

The National Parliament of the Kingdom of Spain consists of two chambers, the Congress of Deputies and the Senate. In each of them, the Spanish electorate is democratically represented by way of political parties.

Future laws begin in the Chambers as projects from the Government, or as Proposals from the parliamentary political groups. There are two procedures for approval: the Plenaries of the Chambers, or Committees with full legislative competence. Once approved, they are published in the Bulletin of the General Cortes, sanctioned by the President of the Government and by the King, and then published in the Official Bulletin of the State.

There are various types of committees in the Congress of Deputies and in the Senate: permanent legislative committees (Committee of Health and Consumption, of Justice, etc.), non-legislative permanent committees, and mixed and special committees.

By the first amendment to the Law for the Encouragement and General Co-ordination of Scientific Investigation and Tech-

---

1. Member of Parliament.

nological Development of 1986, known as the "Science Law", there was created a Joint Commission of the Congress and the Senate to establish the National Plan for Scientific Investigation and Technological Development, and the Annual Report on its development.

There is also a Mixed Commission for the Study of the Drug Problem, and a Mixed Commission on the Rights of Women.

Special Committee for the Study of Assisted Reproduction

In 1985, a Special Committee for the Study of Assisted Reproduction was set up in the Congress of Deputies, which Mr. Palacios had the honour of chairing. It consisted of 36 experts in the various relevant fields: gynaecology, genetics, sterility, penal and civil rights, ethics, etc., who were chosen by the various political groups of the Chamber.

The President of the Chamber was requested to send the papers which had been drafted and adopted by this Committee to other Parliaments, documentation on these matters from the Council of Europe and the European Union was digested and handled, and the experts, besides direct work in meetings, carried out 26 studies. The result of this work was the adoption by the Plenary of Congress in April 1986 of a report with 157 recommendations which served as the basis of the proposals *(see above)* which gave rise to the Laws 35/88 and 42/88. The report was published in the official bulletin of the General Cortes, also in commercial form, and was placed at the disposition of the Publications Department of the Congress.

The work of this Commission and its reception in Parliament stimulated a very full public debate in Spanish society about these techniques and their ethical and legal implications, in which the media played an important role. Moreover, all the written material can be found in the archives of Congress, which may be consulted by professors, graduate students, students and others, who are authorized for a period of one month, and this frequently happens.

Laws and regulations *(Leyes y normas)*

The following laws bearing on bioethics have been approved by the national Parliament:

— **Law 35/88 on the technology of assisted reproduction.** This law has been in effect for six years: its basic aim is the treatment of human sterility with such technology when it is scientifically and clinically indicated. Its fields of application are the usual ones:

• the different artificial techniques of reproduction, particularly artificial insemination and *in vitro* fertilisation;

• the prevention, diagnosis and treatment of genetic diseases;

• investigation of, and experimentation on pre-embryos, that is to say until the fourteenth day after the fertilization of the human ovum, when implantation in the womb has occurred and the neural crest or primitive streak appears.

The law regulates the authorisation and functioning of the Health Centres and Services where the techniques are used, the requirements of the biomedical teams responsible, and gamete and pre-embryo banks. It determines that these techniques may be used by any woman who is in a good state of psychophysical health, capable of giving, and in fact having given, her informed consent: informed, that is, on all the biological, juridical, social, ethical and economic circumstances which surround the application of the technique. Assisted human fertilization for any purpose other than reproduction is prohibited, and the law establishes the status of pre-embryos.

It authorizes the free and anonymous donation of gametes and pre-embryos and their cryo-conservation for a maximum of five years, *post-mortem* gestation, the investigation of gametes and pre-embryos for basic/diagnostic or experimental purposes (in this case only of non-viable pre-embryos under a project which has been duly authorized when the achievement of the same aims by the use of animal subjects has been taken as far as it can be). Substitute or surrogate gestation is declared to be an agreement without force of law, whether with or without a contract, which reaffirms the rule that maternity is determined by parturition.

The law establishes offences and penalties. They are of an administrative character, although the Draft Penal Code contains penal sanctions for certain applications of this law concerning genetic manipulation or improper use of the techniques, in particular the omission of previous and informed consent.

By its article 21, Law 35/88 states that the Government will establish a national commission on assisted reproduction, which has not yet happened, though the Royal Order for its establishment is in the phase of public consultation as a preliminary to its submission to the Council of Ministers, which may have already occurred before the publication of the present text. The commission will consist of representatives of the various organizations concerned with human fertility, of the Government, and of the Administration, and will include a council covering a wide social spectrum. It will be permanent, and will be devoted to orienting the utilization of these techniques, to collaborating with the Administration on the compilation and updating of scientific and technical knowledge, and on the formulation of criteria for the work of the health centres and services where the techniques of artifical reproduction are practised, so as to maximize their utility. In the absence of relevant regulations, this commission will exercise a delegated power to authorize scientific, diagnostic and therapeutic projects, and projects of investigation and experimentation. The commission is expected to be set up within a few weeks of the time of writing.

— Law 42/88 on the donation and use of human embryos and foetuses and their cells, tissues and organs. This deals with the matters in its title, and complements Law 27/78 on the donation and transplantation of organs between persons after birth. In its Section III, it deals with genetic investigation, experimentation and technology, whether with simple or recombinant material, for diagnostic or industrial purposes and, whether preventive, diagnostic or therapeutic, it lays down the functions and powers of the National Commission on the control of the donation and use of human embryos and foetuses.

— **Law 25/90: The Medicines Act.** Under article 64, this Law establishes that "no clinical trial may be carried out without a previous report to an independent clinical investigations ethics committee, and the necessary agreement of the competent sanitary authority, which will take into account the methodological, ethical and legal aspects of the proposed protocol, likewise the balance of risks and benefits to be expected from the trial. The committees will be composed (as a minimum) of an integrated interdisciplinary team of doctors, hospital pharmacists, clinical pharmacologists, nursing personnel and persons outside the health professions, of whom at least one must be a jurist.

Royal Order 561/93 [secondary legislation], by which "the conditions for carrying out clinical trials of medicines are established", develops Section III of the Medicines Law.

— **The Law of 1994** "to establish the juridical regime for the confined use, the intentional liberation, and the commercial exploitation of genetically modified organisms, in order to prevent possible risks to human health and to the environment". This law was approved by the Plenary of Congress on 19 may 1994 to give effect to Directives 219/90 and 220/90 of the European Commission. Under it, the Government must proceed to the creation of a National Biosecurity Committee, "covering activities related to the production, use, liberation and commercial exploitation of genetically modified organisms, which will act as an advisory body to the Central Government and to the Governments of the Regions (*Comunidades Autonomas*), when invited to do so". This Committee will "punctually report on the requests for authorisation which lie within the competence of the Central Government and will exercise such other powers as may be laid down in the Royal Order for its creation. It will consist of representatives of various Ministries, also of people and institutions expert in the subject matter of the said law".

Among the Autonomous Regional Parliaments, only that of the Generality of Catalonia has legislated, with an Order on the accreditation of clinical ethical committees of 14 December 1993.

Ministry of Health and Consumption

The Health Council was created by Royal Order N° 858 of 1 July 1992, and was further developed by the Order of 20 November that year. It is a consultative organ to assist the Minister of Health and Consumption on the work of that Department and on the formulation of health policy.

The Health Council consists of people of a recognized standing in health-related fields: medicine, health sciences, social and economic sciences and disciplines, with an honorary president, a president, a secretary and not more than twenty-five members. It works as a Plenary which meets at least twice a year and it can appoint *ad hoc* working groups.

The National Health Service, and especially the hospital service, has financed education in bioethics, and at the end of the last course (1993-1994) at the Complutense University degrees of "Master of Bioethics" (43 doctors) and "Experts in Clinical Bioethics" (38 graduates in nursing) were created. Almost all these graduates belong to the public hospitals of the National Institute of Health.

A working group composed of six masters of bioethics has put to the director general of that Institute a plan to create Clinical Ethics Committees in the centres of the Institute, with a consultative and interdisciplinary character, to analyse and judge the resolution of possible ethical conflicts which could arise from clinical practice in public health institutions, with the aim of improving the quality of the service.

Ministry of Justice

In 1985, a working group was set up in the General Directorate of Registration and the Notarial Department on "problems in civil law arising from artificial insemination and *in vitro* fertilization", composed of jurists, medical specialists in these matters, and professors of morals and ethics. A report of the meetings of this working group was published on 15 January 1986 in the Information Bulletin n° 3/86 of the Ministry of Justice.

The report addressed a wide series of matters arising from the application of these techniques, such as the protection of the embryo, donation, conservation, different techniques, surrogate gestation, *post-mortem* fertilization, research and experimentation, anonymity, etc.

Bioethics information in the United Kingdom Parliament

PETER DAVIS[1]

Note on the British Parliamentary System (Lord Kennet)

The United Kingdom is a constitutional monarchy. Power resides in the Parliament, which consists of the House of Commons and the House of Lords.

The 651 members of the Commons are elected for a maximum of five years by all citizens of 18 and over, by direct suffrage ("first past the post" system).

The House of Lords is composed of hereditary Peers of the Realm, Life Peers and Peeresses created by the Sovereign on the advice of the party leaders for outstanding public service, and Lords of Appeal. These last, the "law lords", sitting separately for the purpose, also constitute the country's supreme court of appeal.

Draft laws are presented to Parliament in the form of Bills, either by the Government or by individual members of either House. Though legislation may be initiated in either House, most of it is initiated in the Commons. Each bill is debated

---

1. Deputy Librarian, House of Lords.

three times (three "readings") in the Commons, and is then passed to the Lords (less often, vice versa). The second House then returns it to the first after three readings, usually with amendments, which must be agreed by the first House if the bill is to pass. In the event of irreconcilable disagreement, the House of Commons wins. Thus the House of Lords may delay, but cannot prevent, any bill from becoming law once it has been passed by the Commons. The last stage is the Royal assent, which is automatic.

Executive power is held by the Cabinet, chaired by a Prime Minister. The Cabinet is responsible to the House of Commons, and all its members must be members of one House of Parliament or the other.

*
* *

Parliamentary procedures

Parliamentary procedures which may be used by Members of either House to elicit information from the Government or to initiate debate include the tabling of questions for written or oral answer, the tabling of motions for debate, and the introduction of Private Members' Bills (*i.e.* draft public legislation sponsored by Members who are not Members of the Government). To elicit information from persons outside Government, Members may move for the appointment of a Select Committee, or lobby for their concerns to be taken up by an existing Select Committee. Select Committees are committees of inquiry. Some of the Select Committees are permanent, others are temporary, being set up to investigate a particular issue of current concern.

Work of Committees on primary legislation

In each House, the general principles of a Public Bill — *i.e.* a Bill relating to matters of public policy which is introduced directly by a Member of either House, whether a Member of the Government or not — are considered initially by the whole house. If the general principles are agreed, the Bill is then subjected to detailed examination and amendment, clause by clause, by a Committee of Members and returned for further consideration and amendment to the House. With occasional exceptions, such Committees do not take oral or written evidence. Public bills are generally published following their introduction and thereafter, if amended, at the completion of each stage of their parliamentary progress. Lists of proposed amendments are also published at each stage. The proceedings are held in public, and the minutes of proceedings and the verbatim reports of the debates are published.

In the House of Commons, unless otherwise ordered, all Public Bills are committed to Standing Committees for their committee stage. Standing Committees are *ad hoc* committees sitting principally to debate legislation, they are not permanent committees. Standing Committee membership, with the exceptions of the Scottish and Welsh Grand Committees and the Northern Ireland and Regional Affairs Committee, is ad hoc. The Standing Committees are reconstituted and Members are nominated afresh by their party managers for each new Bill or matter committed to Standing Committee. Certain Bills, especially those of major constitutional importance, are dealt with not by Standing Committee but by a Committee of the whole House, which consists of all Members of the House. Since 1980, Bills may occasionally be referred to a Special Standing Committee which has powers to send for persons, papers and records and may hold hearings of oral evidence from witnesses. These powers are limited but give the Special Standing Committees greater flexibility.

In the House of Lords, the committee stage of most Public Bills is taken in a Committee of the whole House. A Select Committee may be appointed ad hoc to take evidence on Bills given a Second Reading by the House: its report, which is published, must be debated before the Bill can proceed. Public Bills of a technical and non-controversial nature are occasionally committed to a Public Bill Committee.

Work of investigative Committees

House of Commons Select Committees include those appointed by the House to examine the expenditure, administration and policy of the principal government departments. There are Select Committees responsible for Health (covering the activities of the Department of Health) and for Science and Technology (covering the Office of Science and Technology), each with eleven Members. The Committee Members are nominated by the House. Each Committee has its own staff and also powers to call evidence by sending for persons, papers, and records; to sit notwithstanding any adjournment of the House; and to appoint specialist advisers, either to supply information which is not readily available, or to elucidate matters of complexity within the committee's terms of reference. The deliberative meetings of such Committees take place in private but evidence is heard in public (unless confidential or classified evidence is being given), and may be recorded for broadcasting. The reports, including the written and oral evidence on which they are based, are published. The Social Services Committee of the House of Commons, which covered the activities of the then Department of Health and Social Security, conducted extensive enquiries and published reports on *Problems Associated with AIDS* (1986-87) and AIDS (1988-89).

House of Lords Select Committees fall into three main categories. There are two sessional subject Select Committees, the European Communities Committee and the Science and

Technology Committee; there are ad hoc committees on specialized subjects; and there are committees for internal administrative matters.

House of Lords subject Select Committees hear evidence in public, and produce reports which are published and subsequently debated by the House. The Select Committee on the European Communities was set up in 1974 following the United Kingdom's accession to the EC. It has wide terms of reference broadly to scrutinize Community legislation. A number of sub-committees have been established to cover key subject areas such as energy, law, environment and trade. The Science and Technology Committee also has very broad terms of reference to consider science and technology. It comprises fifteen Members and operates through two Sub-Committees, each consisting of about half the members of the main committee. The two Sub-Committees each carry out detailed enquiries on subjects chosen by the Committee; their membership changes with each enquiry and Lords with relevant expertise who are not Members of the main Committee are co-opted as appropriate. Any Peer may attend and speak at a Committee when evidence is being taken.

The House of Lords may also set up ad hoc Committees on specialized subjects of general public interest. Most recently, a Select Committee on Medical Ethics was set up in February 1993. This committee's terms of reference cover patient care, medical technology, medicine and the law, and euthanasia. It has reported on Euthanasia, recommending no change in the law. Ad hoc Select Committees may also be appointed to take evidence on Bills given a Second Reading by the House.

Specialist advisers

Select Committees of both Houses are empowered to appoint specialist advisers either to supply information which is not readily available, or to elucidate matters of complexity either within the Committee's term of reference, or in connection with the matter referred to it, as appropriate. Such advisers normally attend not only meetings of the Committees at which oral evidence is taken but also meetings at which the Committee deliberates. They do not examine witnesses or take part in voting. They are normally paid a daily fee at rates broadly in line with payments made for similar work done by members of academic institutions for government departments. The use to which Committees put advisers varies, but the main features of the job include recommending witnesses, analysing written or oral evidence, assisting in the preparation of briefs for the committee and, to a lesser extent, in the drafting of reports, and giving advice to Members during private and public meetings. Most specialist advisers are academics with appropriate knowledge.

Select Committees may also employ specialist staff to assist the Committee Clerks. (Clerks are the permanent administrators of Parliament, its secretariat). Specialist staff differ from specialist advisers in being full-time and providing information generally in the subject area rather than on a specific aspect of one committee's work. The House of Lords Science and Technology Committee has authority to appoint, for a period of two years, a temporary committee specialist assistant. The Committee has made use of this power.

Government and other official documents laid before Parliament

Official documents are presented to Parliament because an Act of Parliament requires it, or at the desire of a Minister, or by Order of either House.

The Government may issue White Papers, which are statements of policy and often set out proposals for legislative changes, and may be debated before a Bill to enact them is introduced. It may also issue White Papers specifically in response to Select Committee reports. White Papers are issued in the series of Parliamentary Papers known as Command Papers, being laid before Parliament as by the Secretary of State at the command of the Queen, although, in practice, the responsibility for presentation is that of the Minister in charge of the relevant Department. So-called "Green Papers" — policy proposals issued for purposes of debate or consultation prior to final Government decision — may be laid before Parliament in the form of Command papers, or more often deposited in the Libraries of each House for the information of members and, through them, of the public.

In the past there was a clear distinction between Green and White Papers. However, in recent years the practice of having a Green Paper for consultation, followed by a White Paper with legislative proposals, is not always followed.

The annual and other reports of numerous statutory or official bodies are generally presented to Parliament, in one form or another.

Party committees and organization

In the House of Commons, the Conservative Party has a number of specialist Committees, including a Health Committee and a Legal Committee, which meet regularly. Every Conservative MP is automatically a member of every Committee. The Committees provide a forum for discussion of policy issues both long and short term, and may be important in expressing changes of opinion within the Parliamentary party. When the party is in office, the Committees may be addressed by Ministers on various policy proposals. Visiting speakers may be invited to address these Committees, but the meetings are private.

The Parliamentary Labour Party has Subject Groups of Members which match and monitor the departments of Government, and co-ordinate the administration of Parliamentary strategy in relation to their areas of responsibility. These include Committees on Health and Personal Social Services, and on Science and Technology. When the party is in office, the groups can put pressure on Ministers to follow particular lines of policy. The Labour Party Subject Groups are open to all party Members to attend. Visitors are invited, the meetings are private.

Within each of the respective party organizations, staff based either at Westminster or within internal research departments may provide private briefings to Members of both Houses.

The Liberal Democrat Party does not have subject committees.

All-party groups of Parliamentarians

1. Registered All-Party Groups are unofficial subject groups of Members from either or both Houses, which include at least 5 members from the Government party and 5 from the opposition parties (including at least 3 from the main Opposition party), and which hold an annual election of officers. Registration entitles the group to use the facilities of Parliament for meetings. They may exert pressure on a Minister to modify policy or influence legislation and future action. They include the:

— Parliamentary AIDS Group,
— Christian Fellowship,
— Disablement Parliamentary Group,
— Human Rights Parliamentary Group,
— Voluntary Euthanasia Parliamentary Group.

2. Registered Parliamentary Groups are unofficial subject groups which also admit persons who are not Members of either House to their membership, but which otherwise conform to the requirements for Registered All-Party Groups. They include the:

— Alternative and Complementary Medicine Parliamentary Group,
— Parliamentary and Scientific Committee. This Committee was established in 1939. It includes Members of both Houses of

Parliament (House of Commons 107, House of Lords 81), 19 British Members of the European Parliament and some honorary and life members. It also includes representatives of: 134 scientific and technical organizations, 75 member companies, 60 universities. Its aim is to provide permanent liaison between Parliament, science-based industries and the academic world. The Committee holds many well attended half-day conferences each year on a wide range of issues: 14 in 1993. It is also associated with major conferences, for instance the Conference on Parliaments and Screening for which these notes are prepared, which was to be held in London on January 20th-21st 1994.

Parliamentary library research and documentation services

The House of Commons Library provides confidential information and research services for Members of Parliament in connection with their parliamentary duties. There is a current staff of 207. It maintains loan services and collections of reference works, newspapers and periodicals, *Hansard*, parliamentary papers and other documents. Periodical holdings include some 70 titles relating to health and medicine, 30 others to science, and 30 to religion. The main method of information retrieval in the Library is the Parliamentary on-line system (POLIS) which is used to trace parliamentary references, EC documentation and other official publications as well as the Library's own collection of books and pamphlets. Access is available to a number of external databases including *DIALOG* — a range of over 400 databases containing texts or references from publications covering all aspects of science and technology, including biosciences, chemistry, medicine and pharmacology. Press cuttings services are available. Library facilities are also provided for Members' staff. The Vote Office, which is responsible for the supply of current parliamentary papers and other official documents to the House and to Members, is also, at present, part of the Library Department. The Parliamentary division of the Library provides parliamentary and legislative information and references, references to non-parliamentary materials, and handles reference and research enquiries on defence, international affairs, and EU matters.

The Research division provides a research and briefing service on the full range of topics which may arise in the course of Members' parliamentary duties. In addition to responding to inquiries from individual Members, research staff prepare papers on subjects of current public and parliamentary concern, including forthcoming legislation. The specialized research sections of the House of Commons Library include a Science and Environment section, an Education and Social Services section (which covers health issues), and a Home Affairs section (which covers legal issues and civil liberties). Each section employs around 8 staff, compiles Research Notes for Members and their staffs on developments of current interest within its own area of responsibility, and responds directly to individual enquiries from Members. It is also responsible for maintaining the Library's resource base of books, specialist periodicals, parliamentary papers, press notices and other public documentation, in its subject area. The Science and Environment Section (formerly the Scientific Affairs and Defence Section) has produced Research Papers on *Acquired Immune Deficiency Syndrome* (1983), *Human fertilization and embryology: a framework for legislation* (1988), *The Human Fertilization and Embryology Bill* (1989), *Aids: Statistics and Education Campaigns* (1989) and *Gene Therapy* (1993).

The House of Lords Library provides Lords with information and research for their parliamentary duties. The Library also supplies material to the Lords of Appeal who sit as the final Court of Appeal — equivalent to a Supreme Court. There is a current staff of 18. It maintains book loan services and holdings of reference works, newspapers and periodicals, *Hansard*, parliamentary papers and other documents. Periodical holdings include some 10 titles relating to health and medicine, 10 others to science, and 10 to religion. The main methods of information retrieval are the Library's own ADVANCE computerized cataloguing and acquisitions system and the same range of databases available to the Commons Library. A press cuttings service is also available. The Library's research section employs four staff and responds to research enquiries from individual Lords. It prepares occasional papers on subjects of interest to the House. The Printed Paper Office, which is separate from the Library, supplies Lords with current official reports and Parliamentary papers.

Parliamentary Office of Science and Technology (POST)

The Parliamentary Office of Science and Technology, which was set up in April 1989 under the auspices of the Parliamentary and Scientific Committee *(see above)*, and funded by outside sources, has been funded by and directly accountable to Parliament since April 1993. There is at present a permanent staff of 5, supplemented by one or two temporary fellowships. It provides Parliamentarians from both Houses with information which will enlarge their understanding of the scientific and technological implications of issues likely to concern Parliament, and has links with distinguished scientists and technologists in all disciplines. The director of POST is responsible to a Board of Parliamentarians from both Houses and all parties, which sets the subjects for POST and reviews all reports prior to their release to Parliament. Short analyses (4 pages) of science and technology issues are published about once a month during the Parliamentary session. There is consultation with the House of Commons Library to ensure no duplication with the Research Papers provided by the Library's Science and Environment Section. POST's Notes are circulated directly to all Parliamentary Members of the Parliamentary and Scientific Committee, and made available in the Libraries of both Houses; they may be purchased by the Public. Notes have been issued on:

— *in vitro* fertilization and embryo research (1989),
— understanding the human genome (1990),

— patenting life (1991),
— patenting human DNA (1992).

Recently, POST has placed more emphasis on "technology assessments", where much fuller analysis of an issue is carried out and possible policy options identified. For instance, in 1992, an intensive review was published of the use of animals in research, development and testing; and in 1993, a study was released on technology and the national Health Service Drugs Bill.

Links are maintained with appropriate Select Committees in the House of Commons, and with the House of Lords Science and Technology Committee, to ensure that where possible POST studies may assist or be relevant to their work.

Organization by Parliament of *ad hoc* conferences or briefings

Select Committees of either House may arrange on occasion for press briefings to coincide with the release of particular reports. Neither House organizes conferences as such. Some of the parliamentary groups such as the Parliamentary and Scientific Committee and POST do organize conferences.

Formal parliamentary links with Churches

In a constitutional sense, the governance of the Church of England, as by law established, is directly linked to Parliament. Before it can become law, a Church of England Measure must be submitted for consideration to the joint Ecclesiastical Committee of members of both Houses of Parliament, and both Houses must resolve that it be presented to the Queen for Royal Assent. Members of both Houses may promote Bills to regulate Church of England matters.

As Supreme Governor, the Queen appoints the Archbishops and Bishops who, as "Lords Spiritual", form part of the House of Lords. The Archbishops of Canterbury and York, Bishops of London, Durham and Winchester, and 21 other Bishops of the Church of England according to seniority of appointment to diocesan Sees sit in the House of Lords by ancient usage and by statute, and as members of the House enjoy the same rights and privileges as other Peers. They speak and vote on many different subjects, especially those involving moral and social welfare. The Archbishop of Canterbury's office arranges for a Church spokesman to take part in all debates in which a Church view is considered appropriate. The Bishops speak also in a personal capacity, usually on social or moral issues of particular concern to them, or on local issues of particular relevance to their Sees. Only the Church of England is represented by Archbishops and Bishops in the House of Lords. Life peerages may be — and are — conferred upon prominent leaders or members of other denominations or faiths, so enabling them to sit in the House of Lords, but not as Lords Spiritual. Hereditary Peers who are ministers or leaders in any church or faith may — and do — sit in the House of Lords.

Clergymen of the Church of England and Church of Ireland, ministers of the Church of Scotland, and priests of the Roman Catholic Church are statutorily disqualified from sitting as Members of the House of Commons: ministers of nonconformist churches and holders of ecclesiastical office in the Church of Wales are not disqualified, and do so sit. Members of the House of Commons may address questions on the Church of England's administration and management to the Church Estates Commissioners. The personal staff of the Speaker of the House of Commons includes a chaplain appointed by the Speaker who reads prayers at the beginning of every sitting.

The Christian Fellowship is a Registered All-Party Group.

Formal parliamentary — academic links

There are no formal institutionalized co-operative links between either House of Parliament and the academic world as such. There are a great many informal individual and *ad hoc* links, including the personal professional and academic status of many Members of each House and the contributions of academics either as specialist advisers or as witnesses to Select Committees. The House of Commons Education Select Committee examines the expenditure, administration and policy of the Department for Education which has responsibility for universities. The Parliamentary and Scientific Committee — a Registered Parliamentary Group — provides a liaison between scientific bodies (including academic institutions) and Parliamentarians (see section 7).

Formal commissioning by Parliament of research by outside bodies

See above.

Opportunities for lobbying Parliament

Any individual or group of individuals may prepare and sign a petition to the House of Commons on any matter "in which the House has jurisdiction to interfere" and concludes with a prayer for such relief as is within the power of the House. A petition must be prepared in accordance with a number of detailed rules, and presented to the House by a Member. No debate is possible on presentation of a public petition; but all public petitions which are in order are listed in the *Votes and Proceedings* (business papers) for the day of their presentation, and later published with the Vote papers. They are referred to the relevant Minister, and the reply, if any, is presented to the House and also published. Public petitioning is a procedure of great historical importance but of less current significance; but it can be used to mobilize opinion and to create publicity.

Constituents may contact their Member of Parliament by letter or in person (at the Central Lobby of the House of Commons or at a local advice centre, usually by appointment) for help with matters for which Parliament or central government is responsible.

The nature and extent of the pressures brought to bear on Members by outside bodies vary considerably. Some bodies may seek to interest sympathetic Members from time to time in particular matters, and Members may be willing to act as official sponsors or office-holders of bodies. Members of the House of Commons acting as paid parliamentary consultants or paid parliamentary advisers, who keep the company or body for which they act informed on matters which arise in Parliament and, as occasion arises, lobby actively on their behalf, are required to record these appointments in the Register of Members Interests.

A Register of Members' Interests is published at the start of each new Parliament. The current Register has been completed by 646 Members of the 651 total in the House of Commons. Members of Parliament may enter nil for outside remunerated interests and 88 of those registering have done so. The remaining 558 list a wide variety of directorships, consultancies and, most commonly, earnings from journalism or broadcasting. Members average about three outside interests. They also register sponsored trips abroad. It is estimated that Members spend about ten hours a week on non-parliamentary work.

There is no Register of Interests for the House of Lords.

Legislation currently in force

The Public Health (Control of Disease) Act 1984, as extended to apply to AIDS by the *Public Health (Infectious Diseases)*

Regulations 1988, provides *inter alia* that a magistrate may, under certain conditions, order a person suffering from AIDS to be medically examined, or removed to hospital, and/or detained in hospital.

The Aids Control Act 1987 provides *inter alia* for periodical reports to be made to the Secretary of State for Health by Regional Health Authorities in England, District Health Authorities in Wales, Health Boards in Scotland, and by each National Health Service Trust on the number of persons known to have AIDS, the results obtained from blood samples for the purposes of HIV antibody tests, the facilities and services provided for testing for and preventing the spread of AIDS and HIV and for treating, counselling and caring for persons with AIDS or infected with HIV. The identity of the patient is not reported.

The Health and Medicines Act 1988, inter alia, empowers the Secretary of State to provide by regulations that any unauthorized person selling or supplying any HIV testing kit or services shall be guilty of an offence. Testing is legal when carried out by a doctor or under doctor's supervision.

The Human Fertilization and Embryology Act 1990, inter alia, established the Human Fertilization and Embryology Authority to license, regulate and monitor (i) any fertilization treatment involving the use of donated eggs or sperm (*e.g.* donor insemination) or embryos created outside the body (IVF); or (ii) storage of eggs, sperm and embryos; or (iii) research on human embryos.

The Human Fertilization and Embryology (Disclosure of Information) Act 1993 amended certain specific rules made by the 1990 Act *(above)* on the disclosure of information by licensed clinicians: the earlier act had inadvertently made it illegal for one doctor to discuss a named patient with another.

The Human Fertilization and Embryology (Disclosure of Information) Act 1992.

The Criminal Justice and Public Order Act 1994, inter alia, amends *the Human Fertilization and Embryology Act 1990* by prohibiting the use of female germ cells taken or derived from an embryo or a foetus, or using embryos created by using such cells, for the purpose of providing fertility services for any woman.

The Legal Aid (Scope) Regulations 1994 extend the categories of proceedings for which civil legal aid is available to include proceedings in a magistrates' court in England and Wales under section 30 of the Human Fertilisation and Embryology Act 1990 relating to parental orders in favour of gamete donors.

The Parental Orders (Human Fertilization and Embryology) Regulations 1994 and the Parental Orders (Human Fertilization and Embryology) (Scotland) Regulations 1994 introduce arrangements to transfer legal parenthood to the commissioning couple where a child is born to a surrogate mother, whereby a parental order may be granted by a court under section 30 of the Human Fertilization and Embryology Act 1990 in respect of a child born of a surrogacy arrangement who is the genetic child of at least one of the applicants for a parental order.

Draft legislation not passed or currently under consideration

In 1992-93, the House of Commons refused leave for the introduction of the Children (Prohibition of Sex Selection) Bill and blocked the progress of the Human Fertilization (Choice) Bill. Both Bills would have prohibited the use of techniques designed to influence the sex of a foetus at conception.

In 1993-94, the Eggs from Foetuses (Prohibiton of Use) Bill, which would have prohibited the use of eggs taken from aborted foetuses for fertilization procedures, was given a first reading by the House of Commons, but subsequently withdrawn.

Relevant non-legislative debates

- 18th March 1985 : Lords debate on the prevention and control of AIDS.
- 21st November 1986 : Commons debate on AIDS.
- 10th December 1986 : Lords debate on measures announced by the Government to combat AIDS.
- 15th January 1988 : Lords debate on White Paper on Human Fertilization and Embryology.
- 3rd February 1988 : Lords debate on World Summit of Ministers of Health on AIDS and to current situation in UK with particular reference to the problems associated with AIDS.
- 4th February 1988 : Commons debate on White Paper on Human Fertilization and Embryology.
- 13th January 1989 : Commons debate on AIDS.
- 5th February 1991 : Lords debate on current state of the HIV/AIDS epidemic worldwide and measures required to limit spread within United Kingdom.
- 22nd July 1993 : Commons debate on government policy on AIDS and HIV infection.
- 11th May 1994 : Lords debate on human genetic manipulation and assisted procreation, introduced by Lord Kennet.

Conclusion

WAYLAND KENNET[1]

The conference

The first conference of the Descartes Society Project "Bioethics in Europe: Survey, Analysis and Information" examined the role of parliaments and the media in shaping our societies' reactions to the bio-revolution. It chose two distinct and topical problem-bundles, each of which touches human life and death: screening for HIV and screening for genetic disease. In a parallel stream of work, a study was made of the arrangements in each of the national parliaments of the European Union for handling bioethical information, and life-science information relevant to ethics.

One hundred and sixteen people came to the conference, and this was about half the number invited. Fifty seven were British and fifty nine were non-British, or were from intergovernmental organizations. Eighty five of the participants spoke.

Four areas particularly claimed the conference's attention:

— the competing demands of personal autonomy and of social responsibility (*i.e.*, of a right and a duty),

---

1. Vice-President, the Parliamentary and Scientific Committee. Formerly British Government Minister and MEP.

— information and counselling for sufferers,
— access of insurers to the medical records of sufferers, and of sufferers to insurance,
— whether regulation of new diagnostic and clinical procedures should be legal, professional or by advice only.

The competing demands of personal autonomy and social responsibility

This — one of the central debates of European ethics for the last two and a half millennia — expressed itself mostly in discussions of:

— What is the duty of the doctor of a patient who is HIV-positive, or likely or certain to develop a genetic disease in time: should that doctor compel such patients to tell their partners, or other relevant persons; should the doctor even do so him/herself?

— What criteria should apply to the abortion of a foetus known to be likely or certain to develop a genetic disease later in life?

Rather wide discrepancies of view appeared between people from different countries on these two points, especially the latter. Germany has anchored its ethical regulation in the memory of great evil; France has passed a law enshrining great principles, which will give rise to much interpretation; the United Kingdom favours control by Authorities exercising powers delegated to them by Parliament. (These Authorities may or may not contain members qualified by their study of ethics.) On the whole, the conference inclined to the view that state regulation under parliaments was indispensable, but not sufficient.

Information and counselling for sufferers

In the provision of information and counselling for sufferers, no differences appeared about what ought to be done, but marked differences appeared in the financial and professional ability of the different countries to do it. No-one thought their own country's achievement was satisfactory: even participants from the wealthiest countries thought that the choice, training and deployment of counsellors should be under better public control.

Insurance

The conference noted the difference between private and public sector insurance. Private sector insurers are governed by the need to stay solvent, pay shareholders, etc, and consequently tend to seek as much information as they can about the health status of people who ask for health or life insurance. Public sector insurers, who function on the mutuality principle alone without a duty to shareholders, are governed solely by the need to insure people and, since they are not primarily subject to the discipline of the market, are not bound always to stay solvent within a market-determined accountancy envelope. Consequently their "need to know" is not market-led, but efficiency-, or equity-led which, in public ethics, is different.

It was argued that no insurer should ever have the right to know any individual's genetic health status. But the majority inclined to the view that it will be difficult to make a permanent departure from the traditional situation, where the individual is generally asked to make all the knowledge he has available to the insurer.

National regulation

The differences in national regulation, whether that regulation is legal or professional, or consists mainly of advice only, were marked. So were the differences within each country between the perceived merits of the present system of that country, and an ideal future system. The probability of an increase in "bioethical tourism", and especially "genetic tourism", was recognized, and so was its double nature: uniformity is economically convenient, diversity is personally comfortable. There are markets not only in price, but also in ethics.

Comparative study of the development of regulation in different member states is valuable.

Parliaments

The studies of the twelve European national parliaments showed that with one important exception all the countries used the same repertoire of instruments to get and process information: libraries, research assistance, permament committees, special committees of enquiry, and so on. As was to be expected, the "standard system" was more or less developed in different countries according to the financial resources each country was able or willing to put into its parliament. The scale of the information-handling process in the German parliament was an eye-opener to many participants.

The important exception was the Danish Consensus Conference, which was the subject of a presentation by Mr Lars Kluver of the Danish Board of Technology. Since the London Descartes Conference was held, knowledge of this way of proceeding has spread rapidly in all Union member states. The first ever consensus conference in the UK, on the release of genetically manipulated organisms, was held in the autumn of 1994 under the auspices of the Science Museum; it was convened and chaired by Professor John Durant, who was one of the principal speakers at the London Descartes Conference, on a subject that a House of Lords Committee had already addressed. The "lay panel" of the consensus conference showed considerably less faith in the prudence of industry than the House of Lords Committee, and wished for more public information and less "trust". (At the conference of the European Biotechnology Federation held at the Hague in November 1994, evidence was presented that, in countries where knowledge of the biological revolution was more widespread, the level of public confidence in the bio-industry was lower.)

Conclusion

The virtually universal judgment of the participants in the London Conference was that consensus conferencing under Parliaments, more or less on the Danish model, would be extremely useful and constructive anywhere in the European Union. So far, all consensus conferences in Europe have been national.

Media

The London conference also considered the role of the media in reporting and commenting on HIV, genetic disease, etc. Discussion was dominated by a recent case in the United Kingdom: the campaign run for many months by the Sunday Times to persuade people that (roughly) AIDS is not a discrete disease entity, that it is not caused by HIV, that there is no AIDS epidemic in Africa, and that those who dispute these propositions are objectively the tools of an unholy alliance between the scientific establishment, the pharmaceutical industry and government. The campaign had been so insistent and, given that newspaper's earlier success in opening up the Thalidomide affair, so dangerous, that the Editor of Nature (who spoke at the conference) had undertaken to refute the arguments whenever they appeared. The campaign came to an end shortly after, when the editor of the Sunday Times was removed. The London conference showed that such a thing had not happened in any other country.

General

Among the questions which, though they did not occupy much time in formal discussion, hung heavy over the conference, was that of intellectual property in living matter: especially the patenting of human genes. The implications of this practice for gene therapy are obvious, and the recent and continuing disagreement within the scientifically advanced countries between those who think patenting living human cells *in situ* makes sense, and those who think it does not, are to be regretted. The multiplicity of patent offices in the world complicates matters.

No doubt finding a solution will be slow, but the Marrakesh Agreement of April 15th 1994 on Trade-Related Aspects of Intellectual Property Rights, which is part of the recent Agreement Establishing the World Trade Organization, should make it easier. It is also possible that the work of UNESCO's International Bioethics Committee towards an international convention on the protection of the human genome will be relevant. Nevertheless, it cannot be excluded that the topic may suddenly blow up and catch some of the European Union governments unawares, and their parliaments even more so.

Recommendations

The final recommendations arising from the London conference will come in the report of the Project Board chaired by Mr. Gerard Huber as main contractor with the Commission, when the five conferences and all the ancillary studies have been completed, and the insights gained have been worked together into a coherent whole. What follows is therefore an advance and partial communication.

Although the London conference did not expressly formulate recommendations, it is possible to set out some recommendations which are clearly in accordance with the sense of the Conference. They are as follows:

1. The Commission should consider putting the comparative study of evolving national mechanisms of regulation and control of bioethical matters in the European Union (*see* presentation by Dr Elizalde) on a permanent basis. Things will go faster from now on, and the need to consider co-ordination or harmonization may arise quite suddenly. The parliamentary side of this continuing study could perhaps be done under contract

by the European Parliamentary Technology Association (EPTA) together with the European Parliament's Science and Technology Office of Assessment (STOA). Both bodies would need strengthening for the purpose, especially on the ethics side. For the non-parliamentary part, another framework would have to be found or invented. This would not be difficult.

2. The Commission may wish to consider the desirability of preparing proposals for harmonization in the fields of health and of life insurance, at least for genetic disease.

3. The institutions of the European Union could continue their work on the problems of intellectual property in human genetic medicine, now that a basic world "playing field" has been established by Article 7.3 of the Marrakesh Agreement *(see above)*, in order to make a European Union position clear to the world. The national parliamentary aspect might form part of the work of the continuing study mentioned above.

4. The Commission should consider favouring the development of consensus conferencing in member states, to be be carried out by, or in association with, their national parliaments. It could also consider experimenting with international consensus conferencing. Perhaps at first, this should be done in groups of two or three countries only. They might be chosen for their general similarity of structure and outlook: Denmark, Sweden and Norway would be an obvious possibility (assuming it could be arranged on a European Economic Area basis). The United Kingdom and the Netherlands, and Spain and Portugal, also suggest themselves as possibilities. It may be that a pan-Union consensus conference could in time be made to work, though the problems are obvious. If so, the European Parliament could be involved.

5. The Commission should maintain and strengthen its contact with the work of the International Bioethics Committee of UNESCO.

On all these matters, the opinion of the Commission's own advisory group on bio-ethics would be valuable.

List of participants

Andersen, Professor Svend	Institut for Etik og Religionsfilosofi, Aarhus Universitet, Denmark
Andreassen Rix, Dr. Bo	Bulowsvej U6, 1870 Frederiksberg, Copenhagen, Denmark
Anionwu, Dr. Elizabeth	Institute of Child Health, London, England
Archer, Professor Luis	Prof. of Molecular Genetics, New University of Lisbon, Portugal
Austin, Mr. Davide	Eurocaso, Gruppo C, Palazzo della Sanita, Via Salvo d'Acquisto 5, Verona 37100, Italy
Banotti, Mrs. Mary	Irish Member of the European Parliament
Bardoux, Dr. Christiane	Commission of the European Communities, DG XII.
Bennedsen, Mrs. Dorte	Member of the Danish Parliament
Bennett, Mrs. Becki	Centre for Social Ethics and Policy, University of Manchester, England
Bennett, Dr. David	European Federation of Biotechnology, The Hague, Netherlands
Bernard, Mrs. Valerie	Centre for Social Ethics and Policy, University of Manchester, England
Botros, Dr. Sophie	Centre for Medical Law and Ethics, Kings College, London, England
Boyde, Professor T.	The Wellcome Trust, London, England

Brazier, Professor Margaret	Centre for Social Ethics and Policy, University of Manchester, England Butler, Mr. Arthur, Parliamentary and Scientific Committee, Westminster, London, England
Campbell, Professor Sir Colin	Chairman of Human Fertilization and Embryology Authority, London, England
Clarke, Dr. Angus	Senior Lecturer in Clinical Genetics, University of Wales College of Medicine, Cardiff, Wales
Clark, Dr. Michael MP	Parliamentary Office of Science and Technology, Westminster, London, England
Ceci, Mrs. Adriana	Italian Member of European Parliament
Corbitt, Dr. Gerald	Director of North Manchester Virus Laboratory, England
Dalla-Vorgia, Dr. Panagiota	Department of Hygiene and Epidemiology, University of Athens Medical School, Greece
De Beaufort, Professor Inez	Medical Faculty, Erasmus University, Rotterdam, Netherlands
De Wachter, Dr. M.	Director, Institute for Bioethics, Maastricht, Netherlands
Dixon, Dr. Bernard	Former editor of *The New Scientist*, 130 Cornwall Road, Ruislip Manor, Middlesex HA4 6AW, England
Draper, Dr. Heather	Study of Health Care Ethics, University of Liverpool, England
Dunstan, the Reverend Professor Gordon	Nuffield Council on Bioethics, England
Durant, Professor John	Imperial College, London, England

LIST OF PARTICIPANTS

Elizalde, Dr. Jose	Commission of the European Communities DG XII
Erin, Dr. Charles	Centre for Social Ethics and Policy, University of Manchester, England
Ewing, Professor K.	Professor of Public Law, Kings College, London, England
Exon, Dr. Peter	Global Programme on AIDS, World Health Organisation, Geneva 27, Switzerland
Farsides, Dr. Calliope	Centre for Contemporary Ethical Studies, Keele University, England
Fertleman, Mr. Michael	Student at Gonville and Caius College, Cambridge, England
Findlay, Mr. Jeremy	Assistant to Sir Gerard Vaughan MP
Fluss, Mr. Sev	Chief of Health Legislation, World Health Organisation, Geneva 27, Switzerland
Frontali, Dr. Marina	Istituto Medicina Sperimentale, Centro Nazionale delle Ricerche, Rome, Italy
Giesen, Professor Dieter	Dean of Law, Free University of Berlin Medical Law Centre, Germany
Gillen, Professor Dr. Erny	Commission Nationale d'Éthique, Luxembourg
Goldhill, Mrs. Flora	Chief Executive, Human Fertilization and Embryology Authority, London, England
Greene, Mrs. Lesley	Director of Support Services, Research Trust for Metabolic Disease, Nuffield Council on Bioethics, England

Hansen, Dr. Anders	Centre for Mass Communications Research, Leicester University, England
Harris, Professor John	Centre for Social Ethics and Policy, University of Manchester, England
Hayry, Professor Heta	University of Helsinki Department of Philosophy, Finland
Hayry, Dr. Matti	Academy of Finland Department of Philosophy, Helsinki, Finland
Hendriks, Mr. Aart	Amsterdam University, Faculty of Law, Netherlands
Hilhorst, Dr. M.	Associate Professor of Medical Ethics, Erasmus University, Rotterdam, Netherlands
Holm, Dr. Soren	Institute of Biostatistics and Theory of Medicine, Copenhagen, Denmark
Honnefelder, Professor Dr. Ludger	Universitat Bonn, Germany
Hottois, Professor Gilbert	Director, Centre de Recherches, Université Libre de Bruxelles, Belgium
Husmark, Mrs. Birgitte	Danish Member of European Parliament
Hutton, Mrs. Ceri	Head of Policy, National AIDS Trust, London, England
Iglesias, Dr. Teresa	Department of Philosophy, University College, Dublin, Ireland
Isola, Dr. Annick	Directorate of Legal Affairs, Council of Europe, Strasbourg
Kac, Mr. Jean	Medical Consultant, IBM France, Paris, France
Karpas, Dr. Abraham	Cambridge University Department of Haematology, England

LIST OF PARTICIPANTS

Karretti, Mrs. Despina	United Kingdom Thalassaemia Society, London, England
Kennet, Lord	House of Lords, London, England : Conference Chairman
Kent, Mr. Alastair	Director, Genetic Interest Group, Farringdon Point, 29-35 Farringdon Road, London EC1M 3JB, England
Kilmarnock, Lord	Chairman, All-Party Parliamentary Group on AIDS, House of Lords, London, England
Kluver, Mr. Lars	Danish Board of Technology, Copenhagen, Denmark
Kutukdjian, Mr. Georges	Director, Bioethics Unit, UNESCO, Paris, France
Large, Mr. Arthur	Managing Director, BUPA, London, England
Le Roux, Mrs. Danielle	Conseil National du Sida, Paris, France
Legrand, Mr. Christian	Association Descartes, Paris, France
Li-Chi Kit, Mrs. Kitty	Nursing Officer, Neonatal Screening Unit, Department of Health, Hong Kong
Lister Cheese, Dr. Ian A.	Department of Health, London, England
Lobjoit, Dr. Mary	Centre for Social Ethics and Policy, University of Manchester, England
Maddox, Mr. John	Editor, *Nature*, 4 Little Essex Street, London WC2, England
Manuel, Dr. Catherine	Laboratoire de Santé Publique, Marseille, France

Marteau, Dr. Theresa	Psychology and Genetics Research Group, United Medical and Dental Schools of Guy's and St. Thomas's Hospitals, London, England
Merkel, Dr. B.	Commission of the European Communities DG V, Luxembourg
Miles, Mrs. Caroline	Nuffield Council on Bioethics, England
Moffat, Dr. Tom	Member of the Dail Eireann, Dublin, Ireland
Moore, Professor Peter	London Business School, England
Mori, Professor Maurizio	Centro per la Ricerca e la Formazione "Politeia", Milan, Italy
Nairne, the Rt. Hon. Sir Patrick	Nuffield Council on Bioethics, England
Neil, Professor James	Department of Veterinary Pathology, University of Glasgow, Scotland
Nicholson, Dr. Richard	Editor, "Bulletin of Medical Ethics", London, England
Norton, Dr. Michael	Director, Parliamentary Office of Science and Technology, London, England
Nunes, Dr. Rui Manuel Lopes	Oporto Medical School, Portugal
Nunez, Dr. Pilar	Institut Borja de Bioetica, Barcelona, Spain
Owen, Dr. Ronald	Occupational Medico-Legal Bureau, 24 Greenway, Harpenden, Herts. AL5 1NQ, England
Palacio, Mr.	Former member of the European Commission Legal Service, Brussels.
Partridge, Mr. Nick	Chief Executive, Terrance Higgins Trust, London, England

LIST OF PARTICIPANTS

Pembrey, Professor Marcus	Professor of Clinical Genetics, Institute of Child Health, London, England
Petermann, Dr. Thomas	Bureau of Technology Assessment, German Parliament, Bonn
Reiter-Theil, Dr. Stella	Secretary General, Akademie fur Ethik in der Medizin, Universitat Gottingen, Germany
Robinson, Dr. Paul	Research Assistant to Lord Kennet
Rodger, Dr. Sally	Specialist Assistant, Science and Technology Committee, House of Lords, London, England
Rodota, Professor Stefano	Professor of Law, University of Rome, Member of the Italian Parliament
Rodway, Dr. Anne	Deputy Chairman, Medical Ethics Committee, British Medical Association, London, England
Samson, Mrs. Eve	Clerk Science and Technology Committee, House of Commons, London, England
Sandberg, Mr. Per	Center for Medical Ethics, University of Trondheim, Oslo, Norway
Serfaty, Dr. Annie	Ministère des Affaires sociales, Paris, France
Serrao, Professor Daniel	Professor of Bioethics, Medical School University, Porto, Portugal
Shapiro, Mr. David	Secretary, Nuffield Council on Bioethics, London, England
Sherr, Dr. Lorraine	Clinical Psychologist, St. Mary's Hospital, London, England
Slynn, Lord	House of Lords, England

Sommerville, Mrs. Ann	Secretary, Medical Ethics Committee, British Medical Association, London, England
Sorell, Dr. Tom	Reader in Philosophy, University of Essex, England
Stefanis, Professor C.	Chairman, Department of Psychiatry, Athens University Medical School, Greece
Super, Dr. Maurice	Consultant Paediatric Geneticist, Clinical Genetics Unit, Royal Manchester Children's Hospital, England
Van Damme, Dr. Karel	European Federation of Trade Unions, Brussels, Belgium
Van Der Poll, Dr. N.	Netherlands Office of Technology Assessment, The Hague, Netherlands
Van Hell, Mr. Rene	European Parliament, Brussels, Belgium
Van Hoeck, Mr. Fernand	Past Director of Biology, European Commission DG XII, Oudstryderslaan 13, 1650 Beersel, Belgium
Varga-Ottahal, Dr. Beatrix	Centrum fur Ethik und Medizin, Donau University, Kiems, Austria
Vaughan, Sir Gerard MP	Chairman, Parliamentary & Scientific Committee, Westminster, London, England
Vedder, Dr. Anton	Centre for Applied Ethics, Erasmus University, Rotterdam, Netherlands
Vestey, Mrs. Georgina	Assistant to Lord Slynn
Voigt, Dr. Hans-Peter	Member of the German Bundestag, President, European Parliamentary Technology Assessment Association, Bundeshaus, Bonn, Germany

LIST OF PARTICIPANTS

Walsh, Dr. Pat	Centre for Medical Law and Ethics, King's College, London, England
Walton of Detchant, Lord	House of Lords, London, England
Warnock, Baroness	House of Lords, London, England
Wehkamp, Dr. Karl-Heinz	Director, Sozialmedizinisch-Psych. Inst., Knochenhauerstr 33, Hanover 30159, Germany
Wilkie, Dr. Tom	Science Editor, "The Independent", London, England
Williamson, Professor Robert	St. Mary's Hospital Medical School, London, England
Young, Mrs. Elizabeth (Lady Kennet)	100 Bayswater Road, London W2 3HJ, England
Zuffa, Senatrice Grazia	Member of Commissione Sanita del Senato, Senato della Repubblica, Rome, Italy

Achevé d'imprimer par Corlet, Imprimeur, S.A.
14110 Condé-sur-Noireau (France)
N° d'Imprimeur : 8761 - Dépôt légal : juin 1995

Imprimé en C.E.E.